A Handbook for Guardians
of Nursing Home Residents
in Massachusetts

Gerontology Institute, University of Massachusetts Boston

Neighborhood Legal Services, Inc., Lynn, MA.

Borchard Foundation

American Bar Association Commission on Law and Aging

A Handbook
for Guardians
of
Nursing Home Residents
in
Massachusetts

Demystifying Guardianship
and
Long-Term Care Medicaid

John J. Ford, Esq.
Editor and Principal Author

Contributing Authors: **Virginia Ames**, **Betty Athanasoulas**, **Jean Benton**, **Joan Boland**, **Jeanne Bragg**, **Claire Brassil**, **Flora Booth**, **Jeannette Bradley**, **Judith Gorton**, **Jack Kantor**, **Mort Kayden**, **Gerald Keane**, **Joan Kelleher**, **Marilouise MacDonald**, **Sr. Jeanne Perrault**, **Jessica Tilman**, **Terry Walper**, and **Mildred Whitley**.

iUniverse, Inc.
New York Lincoln Shanghai

A Handbook for Guardians of Nursing Home
Residents in Massachusetts
Demystifying Guardianship and Long-Term Care Medicaid

iUniverse, Inc.

For information address:
iUniverse, Inc.
2021 Pine Lake Road, Suite 100
Lincoln, NE 68512
www.iuniverse.com

ISBN: 0-595-32714-1

Printed in the United States of America

Acknowledgments

The Handbook for Guardians of Nursing Home Residents in Massachusetts was developed through a two-semester course at the Gerontology Institute, McCormack Graduate School of Policy Studies, at the University of Massachusetts Boston. As principal author, I was persuaded by **Ellen Bruce,** Associate Director of the Institute, that the only way to produce a consumer-friendly Handbook was to use the model we developed for the *Guide for Elders,* which was first authored in 1993. That useful document was created in collaboration with non-lawyers, that is, retirees or younger gerontology students in the Manning Certificate and Advanced Certificate Programs. The *Guide for Elders* is available on the Gerontology Institute's website and is a valuable tool for understanding the basic issues involved in elders' protecting themselves and their assets as they age.

In 2002, **Ross Dolloff**, Executive Director of Neighborhood Legal Services, secured a grant from the American Bar Association Commission Partnership in Law and Aging Program of the Commission on the Legal Problems of the Elderly and The Borchard Foundation Center on Law and Aging to develop the Handbook with the *Guide for Elders* as a model. At Ellen's urging, the course *The ABC's of Nursing Home Guardianships* was conducted in the fall of 2002 and the spring of 2003.

Ellen O'Donnell, the Director of the Paralegal Program at the North Shore Community College, spent a sabbatical at Neighborhood Legal Services from January to May of 2002 and during that time, made an invaluable contribution by drafting the syllabus for the course.

The Manning Certificate students who attended the course were the contributing authors. They identified the subject matters and developed the question-and-answer format for the Handbook. They are: **Virginia Ames, Betty Athanasoulas, Jean Benton, Joan Boland, Jeanne Bragg, Claire Brassil, Flora Booth, Jeannette Bradley, Judith Gorton, Jack Kantor, Mort Kayden, Gerald Keane, Joan Kelleher, Marilouise MacDonald, Sr. Jeanne Perrault, Jessica Tilman, Terry Walper, and Mildred Whitley.**

A preliminary draft of the Handbook was circulated among knowledgeable professionals and their input is gratefully acknowledged: **Mary McKenna** and **Lisa Palais** of the Executive Office of Elder Affairs (EOEA) Long-Term Care Ombudsman Program; **Judith Lennett, Esq.** (Northnode, Inc.); **James G. Nelligan, Esq.** (MEDLAW); **Ellen Bruce, Esq.** (Gerontology Institute); **Neal A. Winston, Esq.** (Winston & Moschella); **Deborah Thomson, Esq.** (Massachusetts Law Reform Institute and the PASS Group); **Debbie Brokvist** (North Shore Elder Services); **Ian S. Oppenheim, Esq.** (Oppenheim & Maire); and **Thomas F. Schiavoni** and **Mary C. McGee, Esq.** (McGee & Schiavoni).

I was assisted enormously in putting the final draft together by my administrative assistant at Neighborhood Legal Services, **Lorraine Medrano**. The final editing was done by **Robert Geary** of the Gerontology Institute of the University of Massachusetts Boston.

All who participated in this effort hope that this Handbook will serve its purpose: to improve the quality of the lives of Massachusetts nursing home residents.

> John J. Ford
> Director
> Elder Law Project
> Neighborhood Legal Services, Inc.
> 37 Friend Street
> Lynn, MA 01902

Contents

Introduction:
Why the Handbook?

Purpose of the Handbook

The purpose of this Handbook is to assist family members, non-profit corporations, or any friend of a **Medicaid**-eligible nursing home resident, or one who will need such eligibility in order to meet the costs of nursing home care, to ensure that the resident enjoys the protection of all of his or her legal rights as a citizen, a patient, and a consumer.

In the Handbook, we attempt to demystify the two areas of the law that significantly impact nursing home residents:

Probate Court Guardianship Law and Procedures

Long-Term Care Medicaid Rules and Procedures

This Handbook does not address political issues like the lack of a national policy for meeting the costs of long-term care for an ever-increasing frail elderly population or the societal values regarding how our country or Commonwealth should treat incapacitated elders. Rather, this Handbook offers a practical guide for those who want to roll up their sleeves and help individual nursing home residents to enjoy a quality of life, as best as their abilities will permit, in their homes. For nursing home residents, the long-term care facility is their home.

Who Should Read and Use this Handbook?

This Handbook was written to assist any person interested in helping a **Medicaid**-eligible nursing home resident (1) who resides in Massachusetts and (2) who meets the following three criteria:

- does not have the mental capacity to understand the nature of his or her medical condition or the risks and benefits of any treatment proposed by a treating physician;

- has not executed a **healthcare proxy document** authorizing another person of his or her choice to make medical decisions regarding care and treatment when he or she becomes incapacitated and unable to understand the nature of his or her medical conditions or the risks and benefits of any treatment proposed by the treating physician;

• does not have a **Probate-Court**-appointed guardian to make decisions to approve or refuse recommended medical care and treatment

How Extensive Is the Problem that this Handbook Addresses?

Advocates estimate that there are thousands of Massachusetts nursing home residents who meet the above three criteria: They do not have the mental capacity to give "**informed consent**" to medical treatment, have no **healthcare proxy document** in which they have appointed an agent, nor do they have a medical **guardian** appointed by the **Probate Court** to authorize medical care and treatment. Every nursing home resident has the right to accept or decline medical care and treatment, and a medical provider who gives medical treatment without authority from the patient (or his or her proxy or guardian), except in emergency situations, is guilty of medical malpractice and violates the civil rights of the resident.

Despite the laws with respect to informed consent, many nursing home residents receive medical care and treatment every day without legal authority for the providers to furnish that care and treatment. Sometimes the nursing home staff relies on family or friends to obtain "authority" to provide care. Such persons are referred to as *de facto* **guardians**, who exercise power as if they had legal authority to do so. Such *de facto* guardians, however, have no legal authority. For some residents, there are no families or friends involved, and nursing home staffers provide care and treatment, which is usually quite appropriate medically but entirely illegal.

Why Is this Problem so Widespread?

The widespread lack of adherence to the laws is primarily due to the lack of resources available to indigent nursing home residents. Residents with significant assets or income experience the benefits of the protections that a **guardian** offers, but indigents needing **guardianship** services are not so fortunate. Nursing homes operate on tight budgets, especially in difficult economic times. They are not compensated for the costs of filing for and obtaining guardianship or providing guardianship services to their residents. Facility administrators are either unwilling or unable to secure such guardianships and hope that they escape criticism for relying on *de facto* **guardians**.

Have the Courts Addressed the Problem?

In March, 1999, the Supreme Judicial Court of Massachusetts in <u>Rudow v. Division of Medical Assistance</u> ordered the **Medicaid** Program (also known as **DMA** or **MassHealth**) to provide a mechanism to pay for guardianship services furnished to **Medicaid**-eligible nursing home residents. Although **Medicaid** promulgated regulations[1] that were designed to implement that decision, many nursing home residents continue to go without the guardianship services that our laws mandate.

How the Handbook Is Organized

The Table of Contents outlines the sections of the Handbook. You may have already noticed that some words and phrases are in bold letters, which indicates that you can find the meaning of such words or phrases in the Glossary of Terms and Acronyms at the end of the Handbook.

Chapter 1 contains two case studies that describe typical situations when people need nursing home care and the problems and issues that must be addressed. The first case study is that of Agatha Adams, an unmarried woman who has been hospitalized and requires nursing home placement. The second case study involves a married couple, Mr. and Mrs. Knellson; Mr. Knellson is already a nursing home resident. Both individuals need to have guardians appointed by the **Probate Court**, as well as needing to secure **Medicaid** coverage to help pay the costs of their nursing home care. The case studies illustrate how the **Medicaid** rules for single residents and married residents differ.

Chapter 2 discusses the rights of nursing home residents. This Handbook uses the term "resident" and not "patient" because the nursing facility is the resident's home. Residents should enjoy the same rights they enjoyed when living in their former homes in the community. Furthermore, federal and state laws and regulations provide rights specific to nursing home residents and address quality of life as well as medical and clinical issues.

Chapter 3 explains the duties of **guardianship**, a responsibility not to be undertaken lightly. A **guardian** is appointed by the **Probate Court** over the **ward**

---

[1] You can read the regulations at **106 C.M.R. 520.026(E)(3)**. These regulations are directly relevant to a guardian of a nursing home resident and appear in Appendix 6-O at the end of Chapter 6.

and must perform his or her duties by being responsive to the ward and to the requirements of the court.

Chapter 4 addresses a question that looms large for nursing home residents: How does the nursing home bill get paid? Finances are an important topic, and the chapter includes discussions of **Medicare,** "**private pay,**" **long-term care (LTC) insurance,** payments from Veterans Affairs (VA), and to the largest extent, **Medicaid.**

Chapter 5 describes **guardianship** laws and procedures and explains what a person must know in order to serve as **guardian** for a nursing home resident.

Chapter 6 discusses an actual **guardianship** petition and the documents needed to prepare for a **Probate Court guardianship** proceeding. The chapter also describes what to expect in dealing with the court system as the guardianship procedure unfolds.

Chapter 7 explains **Medicaid** rules and procedures.

Chapter 8 walks the reader through a long-term care **Medicaid** application, complete with application forms. Chapter 9 offers some final suggestions for a **guardian** as he or she undertakes to provide crucial assistance to a nursing home resident to ensure the quality of life and dignity that we all hope for.

The Resources section contains selected resources that can assist a guardian in meeting the day-to-day responsibilities of that role.

The Glossary of Terms and Acronyms contains definitions and explanations of important words, phrases, and recurring acronyms. Terms that appear in the Glossary appear in bold type in the text of the Handbook.

This Handbook is designed to assist any person or public interest agency willing to step up and help a vulnerable person, namely, a frail elder who is not only sick, but unable to cope mentally and financially with his or her needs. Anyone willing to serve as a **guardian** for an indigent nursing home resident should be able to get the help, guidance, and assistance needed to do the job well.

Guardians will not only assure the rights of incapacitated nursing home residents; they will also improve the quality of life in the long-term care system as they help nursing home staff, **ombudsmen,** and **DPH** surveyors (inspectors) to meet their goal of seeing that the system works well for all.

A **guardian** should organize the affairs of the **ward** and maintain good medical and financial records. Maintaining a journal and using a checklist (see

Chapter 9 for a suggested format) to keep track of important documents will help keep the guardian's thoughts organized, and make things run more smoothly.

A **guardian** should not be reluctant to seek counsel on issues grand and small. If the **ward** cannot help with information about his or her wishes regarding medical care, there may be other sources whom the guardian can consult: relatives, friends, or associates of the ward. At all times, the guardian must use the ward's values when deciding medical issues, whether they relate to minor treatment, surgeries, participation in research projects or studies, organ donations, or Alzheimer's research involving the post-mortem study of the patient's brain. The guardian's decisions must be informed by the perennial question: "What would be the ward's wishes if she or he could understand the current situation and speak to me about those wishes?" That is the challenge of the guardian: To enable the ward to enjoy life to the best of his or her capability and according to his or her own wishes.

Chapter 1:
Case Studies

This Handbook uses two case studies to illustrate some of the issues related to **Medicaid** and **guardianship** rules and procedures. Because the Medicaid rules for single persons are substantially different from the rules for married couples, there are two case studies, which are referred to throughout the Handbook. The single person, Agatha Adams, is an example of a proposed **ward** in the sample guardianship proceedings in Chapter 6. The sample Medicaid application in Chapter 8 uses the facts and circumstances of the married couple, Ozzie and Harriet Knellson.

Case Study: Agatha Adams

Ms. Agatha Adams is 88 years old. She was admitted on Tuesday of last week to the Boston Medical Center after she fell and fractured her left shoulder. She was admitted from her elderly subsidized apartment in Quincy, where she has lived for 20 years.

Her closest living relative in Massachusetts had been a younger sister, Beatrice, who died a week ago at age 79 and who was Agatha's primary caregiver. When the manager of the elderly housing development learned of Beatrice's death, she tried to contact Agatha but got no response when she knocked at her door or called her on the telephone. She called a niece, Becky Thatcher, who lives in Great Barrington, Massachusetts, on the New York border. Becky came immediately and discovered Agatha unconscious in her unit. She had her brought by ambulance to the hospital.

Becky reports that Agatha has experienced dementia for at least two years, but Beatrice and some neighbors have been able to keep her safe at home, sometimes staying overnight. Agatha is not oriented to time or place but does recognize her niece. Agatha needs physical therapy to regain mobility in her arm and shoulder, but she is also diagnosed with congestive heart failure and chronic obstructive pulmonary disease. Her late sister was a retired nurse and she had supervised Agatha's medications until last week. Ms. Adams needs nursing home placement, but she clearly lacks the capacity to understand her medical conditions and the proposed treatment. She cannot sign an admissions contract, and she has become increasingly agitated. She has a **healthcare proxy document** that names her late sister as her agent. Several nursing homes, including the Eveningtide in nearby Milton, have sent admissions staff who have evaluated Agatha as appropriate for placement in their facilities. Eveningtide will not admit her without legal authority; a legal guardian, with authority to make medical decisions, must be appointed by the **Probate Court**.

Agatha's niece Becky needs to know:

- How does she get her aunt out of the hospital and into a nursing home?

- Can she sign the admission contract to admit Agatha to the Eveningtide Nursing Home?

- Can she authorize medical treatment for Agatha at the hospital? At Eveningtide?

- How will Agatha's medical bills be paid?

- Where can she get help? From the hospital discharge planners? From the nursing home? From the nursing home **Ombudsman** Program? From elder services? From legal services?

Case Study: Ozzie and Harriet Knellson

Ozzie and Harriet are married and own a home at 123 Clover Circle, Dorchester. Ozzie is 82 and Harriet is 79. They have been married for 55 years and have two children, David and Ricky. Ozzie was diagnosed with Alzheimer's disease in 1997. Harriet, with help from the local elder services program, kept him at home until April 1, 2003, when it became impossible to manage his care there.

Ozzie was admitted to the Greater Boston Nursing Home on April 1, 2003. Both spouses have Medicare A (hospital insurance) and B (medical insurance) and Medex 3 (Medicare supplemental insurance) for health insurance costs coverage. The new treating physician agrees with the former primary care doctor that Ozzie needs to take the medication Respiridol to reduce the agitation associated with his dementia. Ozzie spits out all his medications and the doctor says that he needs to have a *Rogers* **guardian**.

In addition to their home, the Knellsons have bank accounts at the Hugely Bank, (checking-$1,200.00), Boston Savings Bank (C/Ds—$20,000.00), and Town Savings Bank (savings-$18,000.00). Both have life insurance policies with

Metropolitan Life. They have a 1998 Mercury Sable, which Harriet drives. Ozzie's monthly income from Social Security is $860.00; his pension from GE is $420.00. Harriet's monthly income from Social Security is $430.00.

Harriet needs to know:

- Will she have to use all their savings to pay for nursing home care?

- Will she have to sell her home and move to elderly housing

- How will she pay for the *Rogers* **guardianship** court costs and lawyers' fees?

- If **Medicaid** (**MassHealth**) will help, what documents should she assemble in preparation for the Medicaid application?

Answers to the questions that the case studies pose make up the substance of the Handbook.

Chapter 2:
The Rights of a Nursing Home Resident

1. What rights does a nursing home resident have?

> A nursing home resident has the same rights in the nursing home that he or she had while living in the community. Furthermore, there are laws that specifically protect nursing home residents and their rights, and there are public agencies that enforce those laws.

2. How does one learn about those rights?

> A nursing home resident's rights are delineated in a variety of laws and regulations (to be discussed in this Handbook), depending on whether the issue is medical, social, or legal. A resident has rights as a medical patient, as a tenant or resident, as a consumer, and as a citizen. A nursing home is not a prison, and residents do not check their rights at the door. Experienced nursing home staffers understand these rights. A major responsibility of a resident's guardian is to ensure that these rights are respected. Residents need advocates who will learn about these rights and ensure that they are fully respected. Every nursing home is visited regularly by a representative of the long-term care **Ombudsman** Program (see Question 23).

3. Is there a right to choose one's own doctor?

> Yes, a nursing home resident has the right to hire and fire the treating physician[2]. Practically speaking, however, there are some limitations to that right. A resident may not be able to keep the doctor who treated him or her in the community because that doctor may not have credentials to practice medicine in that particular nursing home. Or, a doctor may not be available because of the resident's insurance or medical coverage. For example, if

---

[2] 940 C.M.R. § 4.08(1)

the resident is **Medicaid**-eligible, the treating physician must be a partici-
pating medical provider in the **Medicaid** Program in order to be paid for
services.

A nursing home is a medical facility but not a hospital. All residents see
the treating physician within 48 hours of admission but thereafter only
when there is a medical necessity or during periodic visits, which may be
every one or two months. The physician is unlikely to work at the nursing home. Care is provided by other medical professionals working in
the nursing home: nurses, nurse practitioners, therapists, certified nurses' aides, social workers, and dieticians.

4. Does a resident have a right to participate in planning for the medical treatment and care received?

Yes, control over one's medical care is a basic civil right for everyone, not
just nursing home residents: The right to be given information about
one's medical condition and proposed treatment, to participate in the
treatment plan, and to accept or decline medical treatment.[3] A basic rule
in the practice of medicine is that a patient must give **informed consent**
prior to receiving any medical treatment. The medical provider needs
not just the consent of the patient, but informed consent. This means
that the patient must be made aware of the diagnosis, that is, the medical problem or condition believed to be present, the proposed treatment, and the risks and benefits of the treatment. A medical provider
cannot provide medical care without informed consent of either the
patient or his or her **healthcare proxy** agent or court-appointed
guardian. Moreover, a patient retains the authority to refuse medical care
even when the medical authorities feel strongly that the care should be
furnished. The classic example of this right is a patient's refusal of a blood
transfusion on the grounds of religious belief. No matter how great the
risks, no medical provider can force treatment on a competent non-con-
senting patient.

Every nursing home resident has a patient care plan[4] in his or her
records, and the plan should be developed with input from the resident

---

[3] 940 C.M.R. § 4.08(2) and (3)

[4] As part of an individual service plane as required by DPH regulations, 105 C.M.R.§
150.004(D)

and any person designated by the resident to participate in the process. Under federal law, the goal of the plan is to provide for the highest level of functioning that the resident can achieve. Nursing homes are not prisons or warehouses, and the resident or his or her representative should insist on an appropriate care plan and the staff's conscientious implementation of the plan.

The resident has the right to see the treating physician, to ask for changes in the treatment plan, and to ask for accommodation of any special needs, for example, additional assistance with any **activities of daily living.** Of course, a guardian has the right, indeed the duty, to assert the rights of the resident.

5. Does a nursing home resident have a right of privacy?

Yes, the right of privacy is also a basic right and extends to the resident personally and to his or her records maintained at the nursing home.[5] Recent changes in the federal law have put additional requirements on medical providers to protect medical and health-related information by prohibiting the release of such information without consent of the patient. Typically, a nursing home resident has one or more roommates; living with others affects one's privacy and creates the likelihood of conflict and the need to make adjustments to minimize or avoid conflict

The right of privacy includes the following:

- The right to have medical examinations performed in complete privacy; [940 C.M.R. § 4.06(1)]

- The right to participate or to decline to participate in activities; [940 C.M.R. §4.06(19)]

- The right to have a conversation with a visitor or on the telephone without being overheard; [940 C.M.R. § 4.06(14)]

- The right to confidentiality with respect to all records, which can be disclosed only with the consent of the resident; [105 C.M.R. § 150.013]

- The right to gain access to personal or medical records within 24 hours of the request. [940 C.M.R. § 4.08(5)]

---

[5] 105 C.M.R. § 150.013

6. Does a nursing home resident have a right to have his or her own choice of food?

> Yes, and nursing homes are obliged to offer alternative selections at each meal and snack, all in keeping with the resident's care plan relative to dietary considerations as well as personal choice.[6]

7. Does a nursing home resident have a right to take part in, or refuse to take part in, the activities in the nursing home?

> Yes, if the resident did not like bingo at home, then there is no obligation to attend bingo at the nursing home. Residents are encouraged to suggest activities that they or others may enjoy. A nursing home activities staff person is very likely to welcome such suggestions.

8. Does a nursing home resident have a right to leave the nursing home temporarily?

> Yes, a resident may leave the facility either on staff-supervised outings or on visits with family or friends. Such visits may include overnight stays, called leaves of absence (LOAs). Unfortunately, the most common overnight stays for nursing home residents are hospitalizations because of acute illness or for examinations or tests that cannot be conducted at the nursing home. These are called medical leaves of absence (MLOAs).

> An important issue is whether or not a resident's bed will be held for his or her return, which entails how or whether the costs for holding the nursing home bed will be paid. That depends on how the costs of care are being paid for. This subject is discussed in detail in Chapter 4: How Nursing Home Costs Are Paid. Until recently, **Medicaid** paid to hold a bed for a resident on a non-medical leave of absence. That policy was terminated in 2003. There is now no payment to the nursing home for non-medical leave of absences. Currently, **Medicaid** requires the nursing home to hold a Medicaid-eligible resident's bed for up to 10 days during a <u>medical</u> leave of absence but does not pay the nursing home for those days when the resident was absent.

---

[6] 105 C.M.R. § 150.009

9. Does a nursing home resident have a right to return to the nursing home after a hospitalization?

> Yes, depending on the length of the absence and whether or not the nursing home is required to "hold" the bed for the resident during a medical absence (see Chapter 4, Question 17). If the resident does not return to the nursing home during the bed-hold period, the facility must offer the next available bed to that resident, who, by that time, may be either in the hospital or another long-term care facility.

10. Does a non-English speaking resident have a right to be spoken to in his or her native language?

> Yes.[7] Every effort must be made to communicate with the resident in a language the resident understands. Residents with dementia often revert to the language they spoke as children, which is a challenge for the nursing home staff. Conversely, staffers whose primary language is not English must not converse in their native tongue while providing care to a resident who does not understand that language. To do so is not only rude—it's against the rules.

11. Does a nursing home resident have a right to apply for **Medicaid** or any other program or insurance that may pay for part or all of the costs of the resident's care?

> Yes, and the nursing home administrator has a legal duty to inform the resident or his or her representative(s) of the right to apply for such assistance, although there is not a requirement that the nursing home actually file applications. A facility, usually its business office, will prepare medical insurance claim forms and will at least identify resources like the long-term care **Ombudsman** Program, the **SHINE** (Serving the Health Information?

> Needs of Elders) Program, or local public interest legal services programs to provide assistance with filing applications or securing coverage.

---

[7] See, for examples, 940 C.M.R. § 4.02(4) and 4.08(7)

12. Does a nursing home resident have a right to a compatible roommate or roommates?

> Yes, although, as in life in the community, there is no guarantee of such compatibility. A resident has the right to ask to be moved to another room and has the right, absent an emergency, to be given 48 hours advance notice of a change of roommates.[8]

13. Does a nursing home resident have a right to be free of restraints?

> Yes, as a rule, a nursing home may not use restraints, whether physical or chemical, to restrict a resident's movement.[9] This issue is often complicated by concerns for safety, especially where the resident has some dementia and is at risk of falling or eloping (running away, not necessarily to get married), or is endangering himself or herself or others. Staffers should be skilled at methods of dealing with such behaviors, including electronic warning systems and personal interventions to "redirect" the resident exhibiting such behaviors. Restraints are permitted when they are required to treat a resident's medical symptoms.[10]

14. Does a nursing home resident have a right to attend church or other social activities outside the nursing home?

> Yes, although the resident may have to make transportation arrangements with family or church members.

15. Does a nursing home have the right to demand that someone other than the resident guarantee payment of the resident's bill?

> No, federal and state laws prohibit nursing homes from requiring that a third party guarantee payment of the nursing home bill.[11] Facilities often require a "responsible party" to sign admission documents, but the liability of the responsible party is limited to the income and assets of the resident. A responsible party cannot be held liable for the resident's expenses but should be willing to explore the appropriate sources of payment for the nursing home bills, whether that source is health insurance,

---

[8] 940 C.M.R. § 4.06(11)
[9] 940 C.M.R. § 4.08(15)
[10] 42 C.F.R. § 483.13(a)
[11] 940 C.M.R. § 4.04(1)

Medicaid, veterans services, or some other source. A **guardian** has the legal duty to determine whether the resident is eligible for such programs and to secure such coverage.

16. Does a nursing home have the right to ask for a security deposit before an admission?

In the case of a private-pay resident, a nursing home may demand a security deposit of no more than one month private-pay costs, according to the consumer protection regulations that the Attorney General's office has promulgated under the consumer protection laws of the Commonwealth.[12]

17. Does a nursing home have the right to discharge or transfer a resident against his or her will?

If a nursing home administrator wants to discharge a resident permanently, or temporarily transfer a resident to another medical facility, the administrator must give a written notice to the resident or his or her **guardian/healthcare proxy agent**. The notice must explain the reason(s) for the proposed action. A transfer occurs when the nursing home intends to re-admit the resident, for example, when there is a transfer to a hospital for treatment of an acute medical problem or illness. A discharge occurs when the nursing home does not intend to re-admit the patient and is unwilling to resume the responsibility of providing care. Except for an emergency medical transfer, the notice must be provided to the resident and his or her representative 30 days in advance of any such action. The notice must state:

• the action to be taken by the facility;

• the specific reason for the discharge or transfer, which can only be for one of the following reasons:

1. the transfer or discharge is necessary for the resident's welfare and the resident's needs cannot be met in the facility; or

2. the proposed action is appropriate because the resident's health has improved sufficiently so that the resident no longer needs the services provided by the nursing facility; or

---

[12] 940 C.M.R.§ 4.05(10). The consumer protection statute is General Laws c. 93A.

3.   the safety of individuals in the facility is endangered; or

4.   the health of individuals in the facility is endangered; or

5.   the resident has failed, after reasonable and appropriate notice, to pay for (or failed to have **Medicaid** or **Medicare** pay for) a stay at the facility; or

6.   the nursing home ceases to operate.

- the effective date of the transfer;

- the location to which the resident is to be discharged or transferred;

- a statement of the resident's right to request an appeal hearing before the **DMA** Board of Hearings (whether or not the resident is **Medicaid**-eligible), how and where to apply, within what time period the appeal must be filed, and the effect of the request (that the resident cannot be moved pending the appeal); and

- a statement of how to find the local long-term care **ombudsman** and any free legal assistance available.

  In short, the law provides that the nursing home may discharge or transfer a resident only for one of the reasons permitted by law and after the requisite notice. [13]

18. Does a nursing home have the right to discharge a resident home without proper safeguards of a home care plan?

  No, and the appeal process described in the answer to Question 17 usually ensures a discharge plan to which both the resident and the nursing home agree and that calls for a visiting nurse or other supports to ensure that the resident will be able to remain safely at home. If the resident is not satisfied with the discharge plan, filing an appeal will result in either an acceptable plan or a **DMA** hearing, where the facility must carry the burden of proving to a hearing officer that the discharge plan is appropriate to the resident's needs. For a discussion of the **Medicaid** appeal process, see Appealing a Medicaid Decision in Chapter 8.

19. Does a nursing home treat a resident differently when he or she goes from private pay to **Medicaid** coverage?

---

[13] See 130 C.M.R. 610.028

No, the care will be the same, even though the nursing home will receive less money from **Medicaid** than from a private-pay resident. Any difference in treatment or care is unlawful discrimination and should be reported to the **ombudsman,** the Attorney General's Office of the Department of Public Health.[14]

20. When does a nursing home have the right to provide medical care/treatment to a resident?

The nursing home may furnish care when **informed consent** is given by the resident, by the resident's duly appointed **healthcare proxy agent,** or by resident's court-appointed **guardian.** The care and services to be provided should be detailed in the individual service plan that includes all medical care and treatment and must be reviewed quarterly.

21. What is the role of a **healthcare proxy agent**?

A healthcare proxy agent is a person who has been appointed in writing by a resident to make medical or healthcare decisions for the resident at such time as the resident, in the opinion of the treating physician and the agent, lacks the capacity to give **informed consent** to such treatment. For an excellent discussion of the healthcare proxy laws of Massachusetts (G.L. c. 201D), see Chapter 3, *Guide for Elders,* at the University of Massachusetts Gerontology Institute's website:

www.geront.umb.edu/literature/guidefor elders/index.html

22. Can a **living will** be used as a **healthcare proxy document**?

So-called living wills, wherein a principal states his or her wishes with respect to end of life extraordinary medical treatment, are not recognized in Massachusetts law. The primary function of a healthcare proxy document is to enable the agent to authorize treatment without having to resort to the **Probate Court** for the appointment of a medical guardianship in order to obtain authority to give **informed consent** to proposed treatment. If the agent and the treating physician cannot agree on whether a document,

---

[14] 940 C.M.R. § 4.03

whether it be a living will or other written statement of a resident's intentions, is a healthcare proxy document, than a guardianship is necessary.

23. What is the long-term care **Ombudsman** Program?

The long-term care Ombudsman Program is authorized to place visiting ombudsman in nursing homes in order to ensure quality of care by ensuring that any problems are either resolved or referred to appropriate authorities. Visiting ombudsmen are trained volunteers who are supervised by professional program directors, usually located in the local Aging Services Access Point (ASAP), the elder services programs of the Commonwealth. The State Nursing Home Ombudsman at the Executive Office of Elder Affairs (**EOEA**) Heads the program. Ombudsmen assist residents with all types of problems or complaints and are trained mediators who receive training in all aspects of the nursing home system. If they cannot resolve a problem immediately, they will make referrals to appropriate resources. Ombudsmen are key resources for residents and their advocates. To learn how to contact an ombudsman, call 1-800-AGE-INFO (1-800-243-4636) or 617-727-7750.

24. Does a nursing home have the right to demand that the resident waive or limit liability for loss of personal property or injury suffered at the nursing home?

No.[15]

25. Will a resident be given written copies of his or her rights and responsibilities?

Yes, at admission. Residents' rights are required to be posted conspicuously in the nursing home.[16] A resident or his or her representative may request a copy at any time.

26. Where do hard-to-place nursing home applicants go and who assists in the search?

Few nursing home placements are easy, but the family or guardian can get help from hospital discharge planners, long-term care **Ombudsman**

---

[15] 940 C.M.R. § 4.04 (3)
[16] 940 C.M.R. § 4.02

Program directors, or geriatric care managers. See the Resources section at the end of the Handbook.

27. May a resident complain about personal care and medical treatment?

A resident can complaint to staffers at the nursing home, to the visiting **ombudsman** or the director of the local Ombudsman Program, to the complaint division of the Department of Public Health (DPH), to the Office of the Attorney General, or to the local legal services program. There are a number of safeguards designed to ensure quality-of-care and life in nursing homes.

28. If a resident requires **anti-psychotic medication** and is unable to give consent to the doctor for such treatment, what is required of the doctor to initiate or continue the treatment?

A doctor must obtain the **informed consent** of a resident for any treatment, and especially treatment with anti-psychotic medications.[17] If the resident has appointed a **healthcare proxy agent**, that person may have authority to approve of such treatment, but only where there is no evidence of the resident's refusal to accept such medications. For example, when a resident is spitting out the medication, such behavior is considered a revocation of the authority granted to the healthcare proxy agent, and a *Rogers* **guardian** must be appointed by the **Probate Court**.

29. Can a nursing home refuse to admit a **Medicaid**-eligible person?

A nursing home may not discriminate against a Medicaid-eligible person in any fashion or at any time.[18] About 20 of some 550 Massachusetts nursing homes do not participate in the Medicaid Program.

30. Does an applicant have the right to information on the vacancy rate?

An applicant for nursing home placement may ask about vacancies or vacancy rates, but as a practical matter, such inquiries should be directed to the local **Ombudsman** Program director who maintains or can obtain current lists of available beds in all nursing homes in his or her catchment area.

---

[17] 940 C.M.R. § 4.08(19)
[18] 940 C.M.R. § 4.03, G.L. c. 151B

31. Does an applicant have the right to have an admissions contract and related documents in an easy-to-read and understandable format?

> Yes.[19]

32. Is the nursing home required to provide assistance to the resident when he or she becomes eligible for **Medicaid**?

> Yes, Medicaid-eligible nursing home residents and those who private pay receive the same care and treatment. Different treatment of Medicaid-eligible residents would constitute unlawful discrimination.

33. Can a nursing home transfer a resident from one room to another within the facility?

> A resident can voluntarily move from one room to another in the facility, but there are rules governing the situation when a resident objects to a proposed move. If the proposed transfer is between beds with different certifications (for example, a transfer from a **Medicare**-certified bed to a **Medicaid**-certified bed), the resident may file a Medicaid appeal. The nursing home must show that the transfer is permissible under the criteria discussed in Question 17. When the beds are of the same certification, the Attorney General regulations at 940 C.M.R. § 4.09(4) outline the circumstances under which a move can be made involuntarily. To challenge such a proposed move, the resident or guardian must send a demand letter pursuant to the Consumer Protection laws, M.G.L. c. 93A. An elder law attorney should be consulted.

34. Can a resident seek assistance for a voluntary transfer to another nursing home?

> Yes, and an **ombudsman** is the most likely candidate to help, since the admission process to a new facility is the same as when the original admission occurred. To learn how to contact an ombudsman, call 1-800-AGE-INFO (1-800-243-4636) or 617-727-7750.

35. Does a resident have the right to assistance in placement at another facility if his or her nursing home goes out of business?

> When a nursing home is going out of business, it must give advance notice and obtain the permission of the Department of Public Health

---

[19] 940 C.M.R. § 4.02(2)

(**DPH**), which licenses and de-licenses long-term care facilities. The DPH and the local **Ombudsman** Program monitor such closings to ensure quality of care during the closing process and the orderly transfer of residents to other appropriate facilities.

36. Does a resident have the right to request a change of roommate?

A resident has the right to make any reasonable request of the nursing home staff, including a request for a new roommate. The facility will attempt to honor the request, although staffers may ask the resident to move rather than the offending roommate. The resident can always ask the **ombudsman** to mediate if the response from the nursing home staff is not satisfactory.

37. Does a resident have the right to speak with an **ombudsman**?

Absolutely.

38. Does a resident have the right to assistance in filing an abuse or neglect complaint?

Yes, and again, the long-term care **ombudsman** is the best resource in circumstances where the resident is complaining about nursing home conditions or personnel.

39. May a resident manage his/her personal funds (personal needs account)?

Yes, a resident should manage his or her own personal needs account at the nursing home or should designate a person to have such responsibility.

40. May a nursing home manage a resident's personal funds (personal needs account)?

Yes, with the approval of the resident or the resident's guardian.

41. Does a nursing home have the right to request donations to make purchases for the facility?

A long-term care facility may request donations but must avoid the appearance that the contribution is anything but voluntary. A resident's contribution or lack of contribution must not affect the care received.

42. Does a resident have the right to reserve a room for special family occasions?

Yes, the resident has the right to make any reasonable request, including the right to request a room for a family function, provided that the facility has such a room. Remember, the nursing home is the resident's home.

Chapter 3:
The Duties of a Guardian

This chapter discusses the general topic of the duties of a guardian. Chapter 5 discusses guardianship law and procedures, and Chapter 6 discusses court petitions, forms, and procedures.

1. What is a **guardian?**

> We are all presumed by law to be capable of managing our affairs and understanding the consequences of our decisions and actions. But a person (like Agatha Adams and Ozzie Knellson in the case studies in Chapter 1) may become unable to think, act, or make informed decisions about personal health, safety, general welfare, property, or financial interests because of debilitating physical illness, like a coma or advanced dementia, or mental illness. The legal definition of mental illness is, "a substantial disorder of thought, mood, perception, orientation or memory which grossly impairs judgment, behavior, capacity to recognize reality or ability to meet ordinary demands of life, but shall not include alcoholism."[20] When such incapacity occurs, and the person has executed documents to appoint a **healthcare proxy agent** or agent in fact under a power of attorney, the person named in such documents can undertake to act on behalf of the person to make informed decisions regarding such matters. In the absence of such written authorizations, however, only a guardian, appointed by the court, can exercise lawful authority to make such decisions for the individual, who, once under a **guardianship**, is referred to as the **ward**.

---

[20] 104 C.M.R. § 3.01(a):

2. Who decides whether a person needs a **guardian?**

> The guardian of an incompetent or incapacitated person is appointed by a judge of the Probate and Family Court in the county in which the person resides. The appointment occurs only after the matter has been brought before the court and a judge is satisfied that the **ward** is incapacitated, that the ward is at risk of serious harm, and that a guardian is needed to protect the ward and his or her interests. A licensed physician must certify that the ward is mentally ill or physically unable to communicate and therefore in need of a guardian.

3. Does a **guardian** have control over all aspects of the ward's life?

> The guardian is in a position of trust, called a "**fiduciary responsibility,**" which means that the guardian's actions and decisions must serve the best interests of the **ward**. A guardian's authority may not be exercised arbitrarily and should always reflect as much as possible the wishes of the ward, when those wishes are known, either expressed by the ward or based on the guardian's knowledge gained from prior experience or from others with prior knowledge of the ward's wishes. A guardian should be responsive to the ward's stated wishes and the input of others who are concerned for the ward's best interests. A guardian has the duty to seek changes in his or her authority as the needs and interests of the ward change.
>
> Tempered by that reality, a guardian has authority to make all decisions that the ward presumably lacks the capacity to make.
>
> **Limited Guardianship.** Sometimes a court will specifically limit the powers of a guardian. For example, a court may order that the ward may not be admitted to a mental health facility without the prior approval of the court.

4. Is the **guardian** accountable to anyone?

> Yes, the court has set up a number of safeguards to require that only suitable persons be appointed as guardians and to monitor their actions to assure that guardians are faithful to their wards in their roles as fiduciaries.

5. Can a proposed **ward** object to a **guardian** or a **guardianship**?

> Yes, as described in greater detail in Chapters 5 and 6, there are safeguards for a proposed ward who objects to having any guardian appointed over him or her or objects to having a particular person appointed as

the guardian. A proposed ward or any interested party may "contest" a guardianship petition. When there is an objection filed, the court conducts a hearing to listen to the evidence (what the interested parties are alleging and can prove by testimony, documents, and other evidence) before deciding on whether a guardian is to be appointed and who the guardian should be.

6. How long does a **guardian** serve in that capacity?

How long a guardian serves depends on whether the court has appointed a temporary or permanent guardian. The court may appoint a **temporary guardian** for a period of 90 days, upon a satisfactory showing that some emergency exists that requires action by a guardian to protect the best interests of the proposed **ward**.[21] For example, in the case of Agatha Adams, her niece should be able to demonstrate to the **Probate Court** judge that she needs the authority of a temporary guardian to sign an admission contract to place her aunt in a nursing home and to authorize medical care or treatment received at the hospital. She would tell the court that Agatha's sister had been acting as her **healthcare proxy agent** but that she is now deceased, and there is nobody with authority to give informed consent to any medical treatment that Agatha needs.

A permanent guardian serves indefinitely and for as long as he or she carries out his or her duties faithfully or until the guardian resigns, dies, is removed for cause, or if the ward recovers and persuades the court that a guardian is no longer required.

7. Is a **guardian** responsible for the debts of the **ward**?

A guardian is responsible for paying the debts of the ward from the ward's income and assets/resources, but not from the those of the guardian. A guardian's own assets or resources would be available only upon the misconduct of the guardian, when a court may order a guardian who has been removed to reimburse the estate of the ward for any funds not appropriately managed.

---

[21] The rules governing temporary guardianships are found in the Massachusetts statutes at M. G. L. c. 201 § 14 and Probate Court Rule 29B.

8. What is the "guardian of the person" and the "guardian of the estate"?

> A **guardian** of the estate is a guardian who has been appointed by the court only to deal with the financial affairs of the **ward**. In Massachusetts, this appointment is usually referred to a **conservator**. A guardian of the person has the authority to make decisions as to all areas where the ward lacks capacity, but such a guardian does not manage financial matters. Typically, a ward whose income consists entirely of Social Security benefits will have a representative payee to handle Social Security income and financial affairs. The Social Security Administration appoints the representative payee, who must file an annual account with the administration. The guardian may or may not be the representative payee.

9. What is a "**guardian *ad litem***"?

> In **Probate Court**, the judge will sometimes appoint a guardian *ad litem* as a court investigator to determine how to act expeditiously in a case brought into the court. The guardian *ad litem* interviews all parties having an interest in the case and makes a report back to the court to assist the judge in making a decision, whether preliminary or final.

> At other times, and usually in other courts, a guardian *ad litem* is appointed to represent an incapacitated person who is a party of interest in a lawsuit.[22]

10. Does a **guardian** get paid for serving the **ward**?

> If the ward has resources, the court may order the ward's estate to pay for the guardian's services. If the ward is indigent, the guardian has to figure out how and whether there are other resources to pay for the guardian's time and expenses. Depending on the nature of the guardianship, the costs may be reimbursed from the court or from other sources, which are more fully discussed in Chapter 6.

11. Does the **ward** ever have any control over who is appointed **guardian**?

> A court will defer to the wishes of a proposed ward if possible, and this principle illustrates the value of having a **healthcare proxy agent** or

---

[22] The court's authority to appoint a guardian *ad litem* is found at M. G. L. c. 201 § 34; also read the court's decision in *Buckingham v. Alden*, 53 N.E.2d 101 (1944)

durable power of attorney document. If those documents, executed by the proposed ward, nominate or propose a particular person to serve as guardian, when and if necessary, the court will very likely appoint any person so nominated, unless the person is unsuitable.

12. What is a "*Rudow* **guardianship**"?

When a nursing home resident lacks the capacity to give **informed consent** for his or her medical treatment and there is no duly authorized healthcare proxy agent, then a guardian must be appointed to give informed consent to that medical care and treatment. A Rudow guardianship refers to a decision by the Massachusetts Supreme Judicial Court, *Rudow v. Commissioner, DMA*, 429 Mass 218, 707 N.E.2d 339 (1999), which instructed the **Medicaid** program to develop a mechanism for paying for such guardianship services for a nursing home resident who is eligible for Medicaid coverage, and therefore indigent, and is unable to pay for such costs. A *Rudow* guardianship, then, is one in which Medicaid is subsidizing the ward's care in a nursing home and is permitting the ward to retain income to pay for such guardianship services. The *Rudow* mechanism for such payment is described in detail in Chapter 6.

13. What is a "*Rogers* **guardianship**"?

When a patient is mentally ill and, in the opinion of treating physicians, in need of **anti-psychotic medication**, but lacks the capacity to give **informed consent** to the administration of such medications, a **Probate Court** must appoint a *Rogers* guardian to monitor the medical care of the **ward** in the context of the plan for such treatment. Under the theory of "**substituted judgment**," the court conducts an inquiry into what the patient would want or not want, if he or she were not incapacitated and able to give informed consent. The rules were first established in *Rogers v. Commissioner, Department of Mental Health*, 390 Mass 489, 458 N.E.2d 308 (1983), and have been enacted in statute form (M. G. L. c. 201 §§ 6(d) and 6A(d)). By regulation promulgated by the Office of the Attorney General (940 C.M.R. § 4.08(19), the *Rogers* case law applies to nursing home residents.

14. What is "*Brophy* **guardianship**"?

When a **ward** is in need of extraordinary medical treatment, such as life supports, amputation, or sterilization, the court, upon the request of any interested party, must determine the wishes of the ward, were the ward able to communicate such, and the**guardian** is bound by the doctrine of "**substituted judgment.**" (*Matter of Spring*, 380 Mass. 629, 405 N..2d 417 (1980), *Brophy v. new England Sinai Hospital, Inc.*, 398 Mass. 417, 497 N.E.2d 626 (1986)) The ultimate inquiry by the court is whether the patient, were he or she able to speak, would accept or decline the proposed treatment.

15. May a resident of another state serve as a **guardian** to a **ward** in Massachusetts?

Although it may prove to be cumbersome, a resident of another state may be appointed as the guardian of a Massachusetts ward. There is a requirement that the out-of-state guardian have on file with the court a document that appoints an in-state agent, who will be notified of any court hearings or actions and who is responsible for notifying the out-of-state guardian of any notices from the court or of any documents filed by interested parties.

16. What behavior would cause a **guardian** to be removed?

A guardian who violates his or her responsibilities can be removed for cause at the request of an interested party or by the independent action of the **Probate Court**. Grounds for removal involve any acts or omissions that are shown not to be in the best interests of the **ward**. Examples of such conduct are failure to attend to the ward's needs, failure to pay bills, or any misconduct, like theft or conversion of the ward's assets or property.

17. How does the **guardian** account for the ward's finances?

Upon the appointment of a guardian over a **ward**, the **Probate Court** issues a decree of appointment and orders the guardian to file an inventory of the ward's assets and income within 90 days of the appointment. The guardian is thereafter obliged to file annual accounts that delineate to the court all of the ward's income and expenses for the prior year ending with the date of the account. All such records are public and may be reviewed by any interested party. Samples of such documents are found in the appendices to Chapter 8.

18. How does a **guardian** choose a nursing home or hospital?

In many cases, geography or medical/health insurance coverage issues limit the choices a guardian can make on behalf of the **ward**. For example, a **Medicaid**-eligible person must be treated by medical providers who participate in the Medicaid Program in order to ensure payment for such services. Where there is a choice, the guardian can make inquiries as to what may be the better or best possible accommodations for the ward. The guardian may consult with family members, hospital discharge planners, nursing home **Ombudsman** Program directors, the Alzheimer's Association or other relevant disease-oriented advocacy groups, geriatric care specialists, or other service providers to elders. The Resources section of the Handbook contains a list of possible sources of assistance.

19. Who can petition for appointment of a **guardian**?

Any two relatives or friends may file a petition with the **Probate Court** for the appointment of a guardian to protect the interests of an incapacitated person.

20. Who can serve?

Any suitable person may serve in the capacity of a **guardian**, and the court will prefer someone nominated by the proposed **ward** either at the time of the petition or in documents executed earlier. The guardian must demonstrate the ability to manage the ward's personal, medical, and financial affairs and, in doing so, has the authority to hire professionals, such as medical providers, attorneys, accountants, brokers, real estate agents, or managers, when circumstances require.

21. In the event the **ward** or his or her heirs object to a proposed **guardianship** resulting in a contested hearing, what happens?

Court guardianship procedures are discussed at length in Chapter 6.

22. What is a *de facto* **guardian**?

A *de facto* guardian is one who acts as if appointed by the **Probate Court** with authority to give **informed consent** to medical treatment or otherwise to manage the affairs of an incapacitated person. Although this is widespread practice in the long-term care system, with nursing home staffers' "accepting" such instructions from *de facto* guardians, there is no substitute for genuine authority to give or withhold **informed consent** to proposed medical care and treatment. *De facto* guardians are not recognized in Massachusetts law, and nursing home staff should not accept instructions from such individuals.

23. When does **guardianship** end?

> A guardianship ends when the **ward** dies or recovers sufficiently so that the guardianship is dissolved. A guardianship does not end when a guardian is replaced.

24. Can a **guardian** who is next of kin order an autopsy?

> Massachusetts law provides that at a person's death, the remains become the personal property of the next of kin. A guardian who is not next of kin has no authority to request an autopsy, unless there is a suspicion of foul play or negligence. Every death is reported to the office of the medical examiner. A death under suspicious circumstances is referred to the state or district office of the medical examiner. The medical examiner investigates and decides whether or not to order an autopsy. If the medical examiner declines to take the case, the next of kin (but not the guardian or even the executor or administrator of the estate) may contact a pathologist to request an autopsy. Pathologists are found at most hospitals, and the costs are bourne by whoever contracts for the services.

25. What is the meaning of the term "**substituted judgment**"?

> When the **ward** in a **guardianship** proceedings is unable to express his or her wishes with respect to whether to accept or decline proposed medical treatment, the **Probate Court** must weigh all the evidence presented to determine what the ward's wishes would be relative to the proposed treatment.

26. If the **Probate Court** appoints a **guardian**, does he or she file reports to or with the court?

> Yes. The reports and samples of such documents are found in the appendices to Chapter 6.

27. How does a **guardian** pay for the funeral bill of the **ward?**

> One of the most important tasks for a guardian of an elderly ward is to recognize the reality that the issue of "final expenses" must be addressed. A guardianship should know or learn what the ward would like to have planned in terms of funeral, burial, or other final arrangements. Guardians are encouraged to make such arrangements well in advance of the need and to fund such pre-need contracts when there are funds available, even if the funding has to be in increments. Because a guardian's authority ends with the death of the ward, by then it is too late to make

any such arrangements. Under the law, the remains of the deceased are the property of the heirs at law. A guardian is well advised to consult with a funeral director for further information on pre-paying funeral arrangements and organ donor and autopsy information.

Chapter 4:
How Nursing Home
Costs Are Paid

1. What are the different sources of payment for nursing home care?

When an individual enters a nursing home, high on the list of concerns are how the person will adjust to the new surroundings and how the costs will be paid. Nursing home care is expensive. According to public officials who monitor such matters, the average cost of private-pay **long-term care** as of November, 2003 is $244.00 per day. A **guardian** must be aware of and attentive to the financial aspect of the **ward's** care and the potential sources for the payment of the costs of that care.

Private Pay. When a resident has no source of payment other than his or her own savings, the nursing home bill is paid from those savings, all in accordance with the admission contract, which will state the daily (*per diem*) rate. The nursing home administrator or admissions director will explain all costs and charges. That explanation, indeed the admission contract itself, should describe the services included in the daily rate and the services not included in the daily rate. A very good resource for assistance in understanding the ins and outs of admission contracts is a publication by the Gerontology Institute of the University of Massachusetts Boston, *Check Your Rights at the Door* (See the Resources section). **Private pay** means that if the daily rate is $230.00 per day, the resident pays $6,900.00 for a 30-day month, usually in advance, and pays for ancillary services in addition to the basic contract price. For persons entering as private-pay residents, the nursing home may require a security deposit, which may not be more than the cost of one month private pay.[23]

---

[23] 940 C.M.R. 4.05(10)

Long-Term Care (LTC) Insurance. Although **long-term care insurance** is not available in most cases, some residents are prudent or lucky enough to have some long-term care insurance coverage, which may pay for some or all of the medical care they receive. A **guardian** must carefully review the **ward's** documents and learn about whether such insurance policies cover any portion of the resident's care, and if so, how to submit claims for payment. If such insurance is available, the financial staffer at the nursing home is usually skilled at processing such claims. A guardian is free to consult directly with the insurer or may consult with the local SHINE (Serving the Health Information Needs of Elders) counselor (see the Resources section). In some situations, depending on the medical care received, nursing home care may be covered by traditional medical or health insurance. For example, a resident who is in the nursing home because of injuries sustained in an automobile accident may have such coverage under a motor vehicle insurance policy.

Medicare. Nursing home residents who are **Medicare** enrollees may be eligible for some coverage of the costs of their care, but the extent and amount of Medicare coverage is very limited; it really does not provide meaningful long-term coverage.

Medicare offers very limited **long-term care** coverage. If Agatha Adams' stay in the hospital is covered by Medicare and in the opinions of the doctor and the hospital's "Medicare Utilization Team" she needs a nursing home placement, Medicare will continue to reimburse the hospital until a nursing home bed is found. If a suitable bed is found but the patient refuses the placement, Medicare coverage will terminate, with written notice to the patient and his or her designated representative. If there is a valid reason to refuse the nursing home placement, for example, when the proposed placement is too distant from the patient's home or family, the Medicare coverage decision, as in all cases, may be appealed. Advocates are available to assist in any Medicare coverage **appeal** and may be contacted through the legal services program in the area (see the Resources section).

For Medicare to pay for long-term care in a nursing home, the patient must:

- be in need of and be receiving skilled nursing care on a daily basis;

- be admitted to the nursing home from a hospital after a three-day (or longer) stay or within 30 days of such a discharge from a hospital; and

- be occupying a Medicare-certified bed in the nursing home.

If the patient meets all of these criteria and continues to do so, Medicare reimburses the facility for the full costs for the first 20 days, and for the next 80 days (from the 21st day to the 100th day), the patient pays a co-insurance of $109.50 daily, and Medicare pays the balance. After 100 days, Medicare pays nothing.

Department of Veterans Affairs (VA). When a resident is a veteran or the spouse or widow of a veteran, a **guardian** should always consider whether there is potential coverage available by virtue of that status. A guardian should consult with an experienced advocate, either the local city or town veteran's agent, a representative of a veterans' group like the American Legion or the Disabled Americans Veterans, or a legal services advocate (see the Resources section). The guardian may also contact the federal veterans' program (Department of Veterans Affairs—the **VA**) or the state program (Department of Veterans Services—the **DVS**). For example, a veteran or the widow of a veteran has a monthly Medicaid **personal needs allowance** that is greater than non-veterans who are Medicaid-eligible (see Chapter 7, endnote 12).

Medicaid. Medicaid, also called **MassHealth** in Massachusetts, is by far the greatest purchaser of long-term care costs in the Commonwealth. At any given time, some 75% of the 55,000 or so nursing home residents in the Commonwealth have the costs of their care subsidized by Medicaid. Medicaid is not insurance but rather a "needs-based" health and medical costs program. To qualify for such coverage, the resident must show that he or she is "eligible" in terms of the Medicaid rules governing financial and medical issues. Medicaid is a very important part of our long-term care system and contributes to the costs of care of eligible nursing home residents to the tune of billions of dollars yearly in Massachusetts alone. The federal government reimburses the Commonwealth fifty cents for every dollar spent on Medicaid, so that Medicaid is a significant "economic engine" of the Massachusetts economy.

2. What is **Medicaid**?

Medicaid is a healthcare program established by the federal government in 1968 to provide health and medical coverage for financially eligible (low-income) individuals. It is a partnership between the federal government and state governments to provide healthcare and medical care coverage to medically uninsured, low-income persons, organized pursuant to a State Plan developed by each state. Like other states, Massachusetts has such a State Plan and has elected to provide mandatory and elective coverage for all persons who are eligible from the federal "menu" of services. A Medicaid-eligible person receives a **MassHealth** identification card and can receive covered services from a medical provider who participates in the Medicaid system. To become Medicaid-eligible, one must file an application at one of the four regional MassHealth Enrollment Centers (see list in the Resources section).

Not all medical providers participate in the Medicaid Program, although virtually all nursing homes in Massachusetts do. For example, a **guardian** may have some difficulty in finding a dentist who participates as a Medicaid provider. Even in the **long-term care** system, there are a handful of nursing homes that are not Medicaid-certified and admit only **private-pay** residents, who presumably must leave the facility once their savings have been depleted by the costs of such care.

A nursing home resident who does not have the savings or insurance coverage to pay for the nursing home costs must of necessity apply for Medicaid coverage. A guardian must be familiar with this aspect of the resident's affairs since establishing and maintaining **eligibility** for Medicaid coverage is the only way to ensure that the nursing bills will be paid.

3. How does **Medicaid** pay for or "subsidize" the resident's care?

Once eligible for Medicaid coverage, the resident must contribute virtually all of his or her monthly income to the nursing home for the costs of the care provided. The amount contributed monthly by the resident is called the **Patient Paid Amount (PPA)**. The PPA is the entire monthly income of the resident minus all deductions or allowances (see Chapter 7, Question 11). Every nursing home has a daily per diem rate set for it by state officials, and each month the facility bills Medicaid for an amount equal to the assigned daily rate multiplied by the number of days in the month minus the PPA contributed by the resident.

4. What expenses will **Medicaid** cover?

Medicaid will cover all services that are part of the per diem rate, which include medical, rehabilitation, remedial, nutritional, and social services. In short, the facility must provide for all the needs of the resident, as reflected in the care plan that is developed for every resident.

5. What are the alternatives to nursing home care?

A **guardian** must be aware that there are potential alternatives to a nursing home placement for the **ward**. Take Agatha Adams as an example. Her niece Becky should consider the options that may be available to Agatha, notwithstanding the pressures she may be getting from the hospital discharge planner to secure a nursing home placement.

The first person Becky may want to consult is a **geriatric care specialist**, a growing profession whose members know the long-term-care system and who are experienced in assessing the capacities and incapacities of frail elders and in recommending the least restrictive and perhaps least expensive living arrangements for the elder. A good geriatric care specialist can show the way through the labyrinth of possibilities. To varying degrees, geriatric care specialists are found in local elder services organizations called Aging Services Access Points (**ASAPs**) or may be private practitioners who are available on a consultive basis (for a list of the ASAPs, see the Resources section).

Home care services. Becky must first determine whether Agatha may be returned home to live safely and securely in the environment where she lived before her injury. Since Agatha's former primary caretaker is deceased and since Becky lives a great distance away, she must figure out whether Agatha can get the necessary supports to return home and live safely there. The local ASAP will assess Agatha and may be able to devise a plan for her safe return home. The ASAP may develop a plan by which a **case manager** can coordinate the services of home health aides, homemakers, chore workers, day care providers, meals on wheels, and other services. In some geographic areas of the state there are PACE programs, which are designed to keep elders who are Medicaid and Medicare-eligible in their own homes and out of nursing homes. Becky may want to consult with the ASAP in Agatha's area, south of Boston, to see whether there are congregate living or other supportive housing programs available to Agatha.

There are also private geriatric care managers who can assist when an elder is not financially eligible for services from the ASAP (see the Resources section).

Becky may also want to consult with the ASAP in western Massachusetts where she lives to explore whether a home care plan is workable where Agatha will reside in her niece's home. If Becky works, there may be an adult day service or even an adult **dementia** day program available that may work as an alternative to a nursing home placement at least for the present.

If Becky proves to be a good **guardian**, she will explore these possibilities now, while Agatha is in the hospital and even later, if Agatha were to enter a nursing home and then improve to where a home placement is a more realistic option than now, given her current medical needs.

Assisted Living. An Assisted Living Program may be available, although such facilities tend to be expensive and are designed for persons who are at least somewhat independent. Some Assisted Living facilities have a mechanism by which a resident can secure public funding when the resident's savings are expended. Where there is no such public funding available, however, the resident will have to leave the Assisted Living facility when his or her funds run out.

Rest Homes. With the advent of Assisted Living Programs, rest homes, sometimes referred to as Level IV homes, represent another potential housing placement for Agatha if she requires less assistance with activities of daily living (**ADLs**) and does not require that skilled medical personnel be available on a 24-hour basis. Rest homes are a vanishing breed, but, where they can be found, they are significantly less expensive than nursing homes.

6. When is a nursing home placement appropriate?

When all housing options have been explored and no viable options can be found, a nursing home placement is appropriate. Family members should always seek the counsel of professionals since many a caretaker spouse or adult child has taken care of a frail elder until the health of the caretaker became at risk. A professional, in addition to the expertise acquired through training and experience, brings an objectivity to the decision-making process that family members or guardians need.

A **guardian** should always have a **ward** evaluated to determine whether or not the ward meets the medical criteria that **Medicaid** requires to pay for the services provided to the resident by the nursing home. Medicaid rules provide that reimbursement will be made only when the resident has met the medical criteria for placement, that is, that the applicant has at least <u>one</u> skilled nursing care need and needs assistance with at least <u>two</u> activities of daily living (**ADLs**). These criteria, called "**score 3**," are designed to ensure that only frail elders are admitted to nursing homes. A **private-pay** resident who is not evaluated risks spending a life's savings only to find that, when the funds are depleted, Medicaid will not pay because the resident does not score 3. In 2003, the Legislature authorized Medicaid to apply score 4 criteria to future nursing home admissions. Medicaid is having some difficulty in implementing such a policy, however, since it is probably illegal to apply a different set of criteria to current residents than to future residents. This policy gives even more incentives to consider alternatives to a nursing home placement as early as possible.

7. What services do nursing homes provide?

Nursing homes provide **long-term care** skilled or convalescent care necessary due to health complications associated with aging, illness, or injury requiring rehabilitation. Services include the administration of medications, special diets, medical-related regimens, personal hygiene care, and general services, which include meals, laundry, housekeeping, and social activities.

8. If the resident is a veteran (or the spouse of a living or deceased veteran), does that affect **Medicaid eligibility** or the costs of care?

No, although Medicaid will permit such a person to retain more of his or her monthly income for the **personal needs allowance** (PNA) ($90.00 rather than $60.00).

9. Who determines **Medicaid** approval for short- or long-term institutional care?

An **assessment** team from the local **ASAP** will evaluate a frail elder in terms of the medical criteria for placement and will determine whether the placement will be short- or long-term. A short-term placement is one expected to last for six months or less. This decision is significant because under Medicaid rules, a short-term placement will permit the resident to retain additional monthly income in order to maintain his or her home. See the discussion at Chapter 7, Question 11.

10. Where does a resident apply for **Medicaid eligibility** to cover nursing home costs?

An application must be filed at one of the four **MassHealth** Enrollment Centers listed in the Resources section. The application process itself is covered in Chapter 8.

11. Does a resident need an advocate to help him or her file for assistance?

> Typically, not only a resident but the **guardian** will need some assistance in completing the **Medicaid** application. Chapter 8 takes a guardian through the process. If a guardian has questions or issues after reviewing that chapter, he or she should consult an advocate. If the **ward** is indigent, the guardian should consult a legal services elder law program. See Legal Assistance in the Resources section.

12. What are the **levels of care** I, II, III, and IV?

> A **guardian** may come upon the term, "levels of care," even though such designations were part of a bygone era. Since 1987, when the federal government passed the Nursing Home Reform Act, **OBRA of 87**, **long-term care** facilities are referred to as "**skilled nursing facilities**" (SNFs). Prior to that time and in some current **DPH** regulations, levels of care terms were used largely to describe how long-term care services were to be reimbursed.

> "Level IV" referred to DPH-licensed **rest homes**, the setting where the resident required the least care; Medicaid does not pay for rest home care; costs of care are reimbursed at the public rate through the **EAEDC** (Emergency Assistance to the Elderly, Disabled and Children) program for indigent residents who meet the financial criteria for either the **SSI** (**Supplementary Security Income**) program or EAEDC. Rest homes are considerably less expensive than nursing homes, but there are fewer of them as time goes by.

> "Level III" referred to nursing home residents who did not require daily skilled nursing care but did require some nursing care and assistance with activities of daily living (**ADLs**); costs of care were reimbursed through **Medicaid**.

> "Level II" referred to nursing home residents who required daily skilled nursing care and assistance with activities of daily living (**ADLs**); costs of care were reimbursed through Medicaid, because either the **Medicare** coverage had terminated or the patient was not in a Medicare-certified bed.

> "Level I" referred to nursing home residents who required daily skilled nursing care, had been admitted to a Medicare-certified bed, and otherwise met the criteria for Medicare reimbursement (see discussion at Question 1); costs of care were reimbursed through Medicare.

13. What are the considerations in selecting a nursing home vs. a **rest home** or other alternative?

> Where a person like Agatha Adams or Ozzie Knellson is placed depends on finding the least restrictive setting and a way to pay for the care needed. A person's health or medical insurance coverage plays an important role in what alternatives are available. Meeting medical criteria like the levels of care is an important part of any such coverage and therefore of any considerations for placement. Consideration must be given to the long term: How long will the insurance cover the care? How long can one afford to remain in the placement? Does it depend on **eligibility** for a needs-based program like **Medicaid**? Beware of a facility that will admit a **private-pay** resident who does not meet the **score 3** or **score 4** criteria; this is a disaster in the making when the resident's funds are exhausted and Medicaid coverage is denied on the basis of a failure to meet medical criteria for a continued stay. Beware the hospital or nursing home discharge planner who tries to find a placement, any placement, just to get someone out of a facility because of payment or coverage issues. Knowledge of the person's real care needs, the rules of insurance or medical coverage, attending to any leveling **assessment** required, and understanding the short- and long-term financing of the care settings are crucial considerations. Consulting with a long-term care **ombudsman** at the local **ASAP** or a **geriatric care specialist** are sound approaches to making such decisions.

14. Is a nursing home required to provide assistance to a deaf resident by furnishing someone who can sign (American sign language) or to a non-English speaking resident?

> A nursing home is required to accommodate all of the needs of a resident. Period.

15. How does a resident use the services of the nursing home **ombudsman**?

> A visiting nursing home ombudsman is assigned to every nursing home in Massachusetts. The ombudsman is there to listen to concerns or complaints of the residents, their families, friends, guardians, or anyone concerned about the well being of the residents. Ombudsman are "problem solvers," trained to receive and investigate complaints and resolve them either by dealing with them in house or by making appropriate referrals. Residents, their families, and guardians have the right to speak privately

to the ombudsman and should expect to have their issues addressed effectively.

16. When does **Medicare** pay for nursing home costs?

Medicare offers very limited **long-term care** coverage. If Agatha Adams' stay in the hospital is covered by Medicare and, in the opinion of her doctor, she needs a nursing home placement, Medicare will continue to reimburse the hospital until a nursing home bed is found. If a suitable nursing home bed is found but the patient refuses the placement, Medicare coverage will terminate, with written notice to the patient or his or her representative. Any Medicare coverage decision may be **appealed** and there are advocates available to assist the **appellant** (see Legal Assistance in the Resources section).

For Medicare to pay for any nursing home care, the patient must:

- be in need of skilled nursing care on a daily basis;

- be admitted to the nursing home from a hospital after a three-day (or more) stay or within 30 days of such a discharge from a hospital; and

- be occupying a Medicare-certified bed.

If the patient meets these three tests and continues to do so (for example, continues to require daily skilled nursing care), Medicare reimburses the facility for the full costs for the first 20 days. For the next 80 days, day 21 to day 100, the patient pays a co-insurance of $109.50 per day, and Medicare pays the balance. The co-pay increases annually.

17. What happens when a nursing home resident is hospitalized?

When a nursing home resident is hospitalized, only **Medicaid** coverage requires that the facility "hold" the bed for the resident's return. Currently, Medicaid requires the nursing home to hold the bed of a Medicaid-eligible nursing home resident for up to 10 days with no payment to the facility. In 2003, Medicaid ended its policy of paying for a limited number of days for non-medical leaves of absence, such as when a resident leaves the facility to attend an out-of-state wedding or funeral. This policy change has put a strain on the resident and the facility when the resident will be absent for more than one full day, since it is not clear whether the resident must pay privately to avoid being considered in a non-payment status. A nursing home resident who is **private**

pay or whose stay is covered by **Medicare** insurance must pay privately to hold the bed during any absence, including hospitalization.

18. What do nursing homes charge **private-pay** residents?

There are no limits on what a nursing home charges for a private pay bed daily rate. While **Medicare** and **Medicaid** rates are strictly controlled, no such monitoring occurs for the private-pay rate. Once a nursing home resident is in the facility and paying the agreed upon rate, the facility may increase the rate only with the consent of the resident or his guardian. The nursing home must give the resident a 60-day written notice of any increase sought.[24] If a resident refuses to pay an increase, the facility's only recourse is to initiate an eviction proceeding, which is unlikely to find a sympathetic judge, absent a showing that the increase is a financial necessity. Similarly, if a nursing home bill is paid by a spouse or other third party and Medicaid coverage is approved retroactively, the nursing home must reimburse the spouse or third party as soon as Medicaid payment is received for the same time period.

19. Who regulates nursing homes?

Nursing homes are regulated by a number of federal, state, and local agencies: the Massachusetts Department of Public Health (**DPH**), which licenses long-term care facilities, investigates complaints of abuse or neglect, conducts periodic inspections, called surveys to ensure quality of care, and monitors the closings of facilities. The Massachusetts Attorney General's office, which has promulgated regulations pursuant to the Consumer Protection Act and which also investigates complaints of abuse or neglect and Medicaid fraud; The Executive Office of Elder Affairs (**EOEA**), which supervises the long term care **Ombudsman** Programs; the federal Center for Medicare and Medicaid Services (**CMS**), which also monitors facilities for health quality and safety issues; and local police, fire and code enforcement for safety issues.

20. What happens when a nursing home closes?

A. The owner of the facility who plans to cease operations must give formal notice to the **DPH** and request permission to close the facility. The

---

[24] 940 C.M.R. 4.05(9)

notice must be accompanied by a closure plan, which will ensure the orderly transfer of residents to other facilities. The DPH and the **EOEA Ombudsman** Programs monitor the process. If a facility fails to protect its residents sufficiently, the DPH and the Attorney General's office will step in to initiate court proceedings to establish a "receiver" to manage the process and ensure the safety and well being of the residents.

21. Should a nursing home resident keep **Medigap insurance**?

When a nursing home resident is **Medicaid**-eligible, a deduction is allowed in the determination of the resident's **Patient Paid Amount** (PPA), designed to permit the resident to continue to pay the Medigap insurance premiums. Medigap insurance, like the Massachusetts **Medex** policies, are designed to cover medical costs (like deductibles and co-payments) not covered by **Medicare**. In most cases, the resident who has Medigap insurance, costing, say, $150 per month, will either be allowed to retain funds to pay the premiums or, if the policy is canceled, will lose the deduction and will have to pay the same $150 to the nursing home as part of the PPA.

A resident with a spouse at home, however, may want to cancel the Medigap insurance if it will result in an increased monthly **community spouse resource allowance** to the spouse at home.

22. Should a nursing home resident's home be preserved?

Certainly, if the resident has been assessed as a short-term stay, the home, whether rented or owned, should be preserved. **Medicaid** recognizes the reality of the situation by permitting the Medicaid-eligible, short-stay resident to retain income to pay the costs of maintaining the home so that there will be a home to return to at the end of the short stay. For long-term placements, a rental situation may not be possible to maintain unless there are family members residing there. If the long-term resident owns the home, considerations include whether there are family members residing in the home, whether there are family members to whom the resident may be permitted to transfer title to the home, or whether the home should be sold or converted to a rental income-producing **asset** in order to generate the funds needed to pay the costs of maintaining the house and supporting the resident's stay. Such a resident or the **guardian** should consult an elder law attorney to understand all of the options before choosing.

Chapter 5:
Guardianship Law and Procedures

1. What is a guardian?

> A **guardian** is appointed by the **Probate Court** to mange the affairs of a **ward**, that is, a person who is, by reason of mental illness or other physical or mental disability, unable to take care of him- or herself or his or her affairs, and who is at risk of serious harm as a result of such incapacity. Our society values the autonomy of an individual and the right to control our own lives and destinies, and the court recognizes this reality. **Guardianships** are not taken or appointed lightly, so that a ward is not placed under a guardianship for bad judgment or eccentric behavior, but solely on the legal basis described above. The guardianship statutory law is found at G.L. c. 201.

> Under Massachusetts law, all adult persons 18 years of age or older are presumed to be competent and capable of caring for themselves and managing their affairs. The power to make decisions for one's self, one's autonomy, may be taken away only by a court and only when a judge decides that, for the person's safety and well being, another person should be appointed as guardian.

> A person who has been found to be unable to manage his or her affairs is termed "**incompetent**" under our current system. The term "**incapacitated**" is gaining ground as a more respectful and accurate expression to describe the person over whom a guardian is appointed. To make a determination of incompetence or incapacity, a judge will consider all the ways in which the person may need help as well as the ways in which she or he is able to maintain his or her independence. A decree of guardianship should limit the authority of the guardian only to those areas where a judge has found the person to be unable to manage his or her affairs and where assistance is needed to keep the person safe. For example, if the proposed ward's incapacities are found by the court to relate only to

financial matters, the court will appoint a **conservator**, or guardian of the estate of the ward, and not a guardian of the person.

A guardian appointed to manage the medical treatment of the ward has authority to manage the usual and customary medical needs and should seek specific authority from the court for any unusual or extraordinary treatments, such as the administration of **anti-psychotic medications**, amputations, life supports, abortion, or sterilization. Where **extraordinary medical treatment** is being proposed, the guardian is required to seek authority under the "**substituted judgement**" concept, where the court must determine that the patient, if competent, would consent to such proposed treatment.

A guardian is appointed to a fiduciary position, that is, one requiring a very high degree of trust, honesty, responsibility, loyalty, and care for the ward's well being. It is a role not to be taken lightly; the demands on a guardian come from society as well as from the needs of the ward.

2. Who decides whether or not a person needs a **guardian**?

In the case of a disabled nursing home resident or a frail elder in need of such a placement, a judge of the **Probate Court** makes the decision that an individual must have a guardian.

There is a procedure available in the District Court where an individual, elderly or otherwise, who is a danger to himself or to others may require involuntary commitment to a mental health facility. A long-term guardianship, however, is in the province of the Probate Court for the county in which the individual resides. The Resources section has a listing of all Probate Courts.

3. How does a **guardian** get appointed?

The first step in the process of having a guardian appointed is the filing of a petition for the appointment of a guardian over a **ward** who is alleged to be in need of such protection. The petition identifies (1) the allegedly **incapacitated** person, (2) the persons who are the petitioners (asking the court to act), (3) all interested parties, and (4) the person(s) whom the petitioners would like to see the court appoint as guardian(s).

The petition must be accompanied by a number of other documents: a medical certification from the treating physician of the proposed ward, a bond form, and a filing fee.

Filing the petition begins the procedure that is described in full detail in Chapter 6 and that may result in the appointment of a guardian.

4. Who can petition for the appointment of a **guardian**?

A parent, two or more relatives or friends, or certain non-profit corporations or state agencies whose functions include public protection may petition for the appointment of a guardian.

5. Who must be given notice that a petition has been filed?

When a petition is properly filed and reviewed by court personnel, the court will issue a "citation," which will instruct the petitioners about how to give notice of their petition to all interested parties (see Chapter 6 Appendix J for a sample citation). A copy of the citation and petition must be given to (served on) the proposed **ward** by a disinterested party, such as a constable, and a copy must be served on all of the heirs of the proposed ward. The heirs are those persons who would share in the estate of the proposed ward if he or she were to die without a will. A person who dies without a will is described as having died "**intestate**," and there is a statute that prescribes how the estate will be distributed to the decedent's next of kin. (G.L. c. 190 § 1: law of intestate succession: (see Chapter 6 Appendix A-1) The court may require that the citation be published in a newspaper, all of which is designed to protect the integrity of the court's ultimate ruling: The judge will want to hear testimony from any person interested in the well being of the proposed ward, whether in support of, or opposed to, the petition.

6. Why is a bond necessary and what are "**sureties**"?

Anyone appointed as a **guardian** will have access to and control over the **assets** and income of the **ward**. Consequently, the guardian must be shown to be a person who can be trusted to see to the well being of the ward. Even the most talented judge cannot look at a person or examine a signature and tell whether that person has the reputation and wherewithal to serve as a guardian. The guardian must sign a bond in the amount equal to 150% of the estimated value of the proposed ward's estate (not including the value of any real estate). If the guardian, once appointed, is guilty of some wrongdoing and causes a financial loss to the ward's estate, the guardian can be sued on the bond and will be required to reimburse the ward's estate from his or her own resources. Sureties are persons who express confidence in the integrity of the guardian by, in essence, guaranteeing to the court that the guardian will be an honest steward. A surety can be sued on the bond if the guardian absconds or is otherwise unable to reimburse the ward's estate if ordered to do so by the court. The court may also order corporate sureties, that is, a bond issued or endorsed by an insurance company; the guardian must obtain a corporate bond by demonstrating to the insurance company the honesty and financial capacity to abide by the **fiduciary responsibilities** of a guardian, since the insurance company would be liable on the bond for any financial wrongdoing of the guardian.

7. What happens if the **ward** does not have the funds even to pay the filing fee?

There is no filing fee when the ward has assets of less than $100. Massachusetts has a statute that permits indigents access to the courts by requiring that courts waive any filing fees or court costs when the party can show an inability to pay such fees or costs (see Chapter 6 Appendix B for information and a sample affidavit of indigence).

8. What is a **guardian** *ad litem*?

A guardian *ad litem* is *not* a guardian, but rather a person, usually an attorney, whom the court appoints to investigate the facts of a case where there is an alleged need for speedy action by the court because a delay may harm any party to the proceedings, and/or where there is some conflict among the parties. Suppose Becky files a petition for appointment of herself as Agatha Adam's guardian, and another nephew appears and alleges that Becky is unsuitable because she has stolen Agatha's funds in the past. Few **Probate Court** judges can promptly schedule a hearing to listen to the evidence from both sides, so the court may appoint a guardian *ad litem* to investigate the facts surrounding the allegations and determine whether the nephew's allegations are sufficient or delusional or somewhere in between. The guardian *ad litem* prepares a report of his or her findings, which is filed with the court and distributed to the parties. If the matter is unresolved, that issue is heard by the court. Ultimately, the judge will decide what is to be done.

9. Does the court appoint an attorney for the proposed **ward**?

Although there is a Massachusetts Supreme Judicial Court rule[25] that says that in every **guardianship** petition, the **Probate Court** must

---

[25] Supreme Judicial Court Rule 3:10 (5)

appoint counsel for any proposed ward, such appointments are not made in every case. Whether to avoid unnecessary spending of either the proposed ward's funds or the public funds of the state, or for other considerations, the Probate Courts will appoint counsel for the ward only if there is a reason for doing so, for example, if any interested party requested such an appointment, if the proposed ward objects to the petition, or if the nature of the proceedings require it. In a **Rogers guardianship** proceeding, the court will always appoint counsel for the proposed ward.

10. What happens if the proposed **ward**, or anyone else, objects to the petition?

The purpose of the rule that requires that the citation be served on all interested parties, and perhaps even published in a newspaper, is to ensure that anyone knowing of any valid reason why the petition should not be allowed by the court will learn that the petition has been filed. The citation informs all parties served, and the world in a newspaper legal notice publication, that a petition has been filed by Becky Thatcher in the Norfolk County Probate Court Docket No. such-and-such, for the appointment of a guardian for Agatha Adams and says that anyone objecting must file his or her appearance by a date certain, called the "return day." If any person files an objection or even an appearance on or before the return day, nothing will happen; no guardian will be appointed until there has been a hearing on the substance of the objection. After the return day has passed, any interested party may file a motion to bring the case before the court for an order giving relief to the moving party. For example, Becky may file a motion that says, in essence, that she needs emergency authority as temporary guardian to admit Agatha to a nursing home, and her cousin's allegations of larceny are bogus. The court will hear from all sides, including any guardian *ad litem* report, and decide whether the temporary relief should be granted or denied.

When there is an objection, the court will order a full hearing on the merits of the petition and will hear evidence from the proponents and the opponents of the petitioner's request.

If no objections or appearances are filed by the return day and the proceedings do not require that an attorney be appointed for the proposed ward, the court will automatically appoint the guardian nominated in the petition, after having approved the bond.

11. What happens if no one is available to serve as **guardian**?

> This is a frequent scenario and one of the reasons for preparing this Handbook. Many situations arise in the community and in the long-term care system where an individual clearly needs a guardian, but no one is willing or available to serve.
>
> Suppose Becky were unwilling to get involved and Agatha had no other living relatives or friends. Since the hospital needs to move her out of their care and into a more appropriate care setting, the burden falls on the hospital staff to arrange for a lawful discharge. Only a guardian can lawfully authorize medical care and sign the documents associated with Agatha's placement in the nursing home. The hospital discharge planners can contact their legal department for help. Their lawyer can draft the guardianship petition and list no relatives, but then must nominate someone to serve as guardian. The attorney can take a chance and leave that part of the petition blank, hoping that the court can find some attorney willing to serve *pro bono publico*, that is, in the public interest without charging fees or costs, but many **Probate Courts** have no capacity to draft attorneys involuntarily for such responsibilities. When the proposed **ward** is indigent and there are no **assets** to compensate those willing to help, there is a significant dilemma for the courts: How can a guardianship system work for low-income **incapacitated** persons if there are only unpaid volunteers? Some courts succeed in persuading attorneys to take cases involving indigent wards *pro bono* as a recognition of the obligation to provide free service to indigents and as a kind of payback for the compensation they receive in representing wards who are better off financially. In some instances, frail elders go without proper care and without adequate supports.
>
> In the case of an indigent nursing home resident who needs a guardian, at least there is a mechanism for paying the costs of needed guardianship services if a guardian can be found.

12. How are **guardians** paid for their services?

> If the **ward** has significant **assets** or income, the court will order that reasonable costs of establishing the guardianship and of providing the needed ongoing services of the guardian to the ward may be paid for out of the ward's income or assets. A guardian must file an inventory of the ward's assets within 90 days of appointment and must file annual accounts with the court that detail the ward's income and expenses. The

court must approve the accounts. When a ward has assets, the account will reflect payment to the guardian, and the court will approve reasonable expenditures.

When there are no assets in the ward's estate, there is no mechanism for payment unless the Court is mandated to pay for such costs, as in the case of **Roger's guardians** who monitor care plans involving the administration of **anti-psychotic medications**.

While there is no mechanism for paying for guardianship costs for indigent elders in the community, the *Rudow* decision has resulted in a way for some guardians of nursing home residents to be compensated for their services.

13. How is a *Rudow* **guardian** paid?

A *Rudow* **guardianship** refers simply to a case where the ward is a nursing home resident who is or will be eligible for **Medicaid** coverage, and the costs of providing guardianship service may be paid from the ward's monthly income.

Prior to the *Rudow* decision, Medicaid took the position that guardianship costs were neither medical nor remedial expenses and therefore could not be allowed as a deduction from income in computing the resident's **Patient Paid Amount** (PPA) under the allowance for "Health Care Coverage and Other Incurred Expenses" found at 130 C.M.R. 520.126 (E). The *Rudow* court ruled that a medical guardian was an essential pre-requisite for providing any medical care to a resident unable to give **informed consent** to treatment, and therefore, Medicaid must allow a medical or remedial deduction for such care. The court left it to Medicaid to develop the regulations to implement the decision. Those regulations are found at 130 C.M.R. 520.026(E)(3), and they permit a deduction where a medical guardianship is established and a Medicaid application filed on behalf of a nursing home resident (see Chapter 6, Appendix O).

The procedure to be followed is for the guardian, once appointed, to obtain the **Probate Court** judge's approval of the expenses associated with securing the guardianship and of the anticipated costs of the guardians in providing services over the next year, then submitting the court's approved expenses to the Medicaid office. Medicaid will then approve the amount to be recovered by the guardian and reduce the PPA for the resident for each month over the next 12-month period by one-twelfth of the amount approved. The guardian will then be able to use the income saved by the deduction, rather than pay the nursing home, to apply it to guardianship-related costs.

Suppose Becky went to the Probate Court and obtained a guardianship for Agatha, and incurred costs of $1,440.00, which were approved by the Probate Court for submission to Medicaid. The Probate Court will approve out-of-pocket expenses and reasonable compensation for the guardian in prosecuting the petition.(Medicaid will also allow a PPA deduction for up to 24 hours per year at up to $50.00 per hour for payment for the guardian, upon an affidavit from the guardian.) Medicaid will issue a decision that reduces Agatha's PPA by one-twelfth of the amount approved or $120.00. For the next 12 months, then, Becky will be able to retain $120.00 each month to recoup the guardianship expenses. Since guardians have a duty to file an annual account, Becky can use that occasion every year to renew her request for payment of costs associated with functions as her aunt's guardian.

Critics point to a number of drawbacks in the Medicaid regulations implementing the Rudow decision:

- The guardian has no recourse if he or she pays the expenses "up front" and the ward dies before the funds are recouped via the PPA deduction;

- The limits that Medicaid placed on the amount of reimbursement is unrealistically low: $500.00 for a guardianship petition and $750.00 for "more complex" cases. The limits are a disincentive to lawyers to accept such cases; there is a provision for hardship, which may allow larger expenses;

- There is no allowance for travel or transportation costs;

- No guardianship costs deduction is permitted when the guardian is the spouse, parent, sibling, or child of the ward; and

- For a nursing home resident whose income consists entirely of an SSI personal needs allowance of $60.00 per month, there is no Patient Paid Amount and, therefore, no way to reimburse a guardian for services or out-of-pocket expenses.

14. How does a **guardian** make medical decisions?

> Once appointed, the guardian should base all medical decisions on the wishes of the **ward** if the ward were able to state those wishes. A guardian who has known the ward is better equipped to have knowledge of what the ward would want in terms of medical care, but even a guardian who is a virtual stranger to the ward has the duty to learn from any and all available sources what the ward's wishes are or would be relative to medical care. Due diligence must be given to the input of medical providers, and attendance at the quarterly care plan meetings is essential and is even mandated under the **Medicaid** regulations (130 C.M.R. 520.026(3)(d)(iii)); see Chapter 6, Appendix O.

15. What behavior would cause a **guardian** to be removed?

> Any omission committed or action taken by a guardian that is not in the best interests of the **ward** is grounds for the removal of the guardian. A guardian is held to a very high standard of honesty and loyalty to the ward and, as a fiduciary, must be attentive to the ward and to the ward's affairs.

16. Can the court appoint co-guardians?

> Yes, the **Probate Court** has authority to appoint co-guardians, although, like having two captains of a ship, it may not always be a good idea, unless the individuals involved are able to work cooperatively.

17. What can an interested person do who suspects that a **guardian** is acting improperly?

> Any interested person can bring a guardian's suspected misconduct to the court's attention by submitting a statement of facts relative to the alleged misconduct and a statement of the evidence to support the allegation. If the ward has an attorney or if a **guardian** *ad litem* has been appointed by the court, complaints can be addressed to them.

18. What is the remedy of a family member who disagrees with the actions of a **guardian**?

> Unless the disagreement involves a breach of the guardian's duties, a family member can only try to persuade the guardian to his or her point of view. A good guardian should welcome the advice of any person concerned about the welfare of the **ward**.

19. Does a **guardian** need special knowledge or training?

> There are currently no training programs for guardians in Massachusetts, although other jurisdictions offer various training books, pamphlets, or videos. Knowledge of the ward and his or her wishes, respect for those wishes, common sense, and honesty will take a guardian far as the lessons of the tasks at hand are learned.

Chapter 6:
Guardianship Petitions and
Court Proceedings

When it is clear that an individual must have a **guardian** with authority to give informed consent to recommended medical care or treatment, someone must make the necessary preparations. Where there are resources available, that is, where the individual has an estate (**assets**), a prospective guardian would be well advised to consult with an elder law attorney who is experienced in guardianship matters. Where the individual **ward** has little or no resources, any party interested in the welfare of the proposed ward may undertake to begin the process of securing the protections of a guardian for the individual.

This chapter takes the reader through the guardianship process, including how the guardian may be compensated through the *Rudow* procedure (130 C.M.R. 520.026(E)(3); see Appendix 6-O) for the services to be provided to the ward. The appendices to this Chapter contain forms filled out as if Rebecca Thatcher were petitioning to become guardian for her aunt, Agatha Adams. Given that many nursing home residents are treated with **anti-psychotic medications** to treat the symptoms associated with dementia (e.g., agitation, combativeness, delusional thought), the petition will be asking the court for authority to authorize the use of anti-psychotic medications as part of an approved treatment plan, which is the essence of a *Rogers* guardianship.

In preparing the petition to be filed with the **Probate Court**, the prospective guardian should be aware of all documents that are typically generated in the course of the proceedings:

Documents potentially developed prior to filing:

- The Petition

- Affidavit of Indigency

- The medical certificate[26]

- The bond form

- Motion for appointment of Temporary Guardian

- Affidavit for Temporary Guardianship

- Physician's Affidavit and Treatment Plan

- Temporary Decree of Guardianship

- Motion for appointment of a guardian ad litem

- Motion for appointment of counsel for the proposed ward

Documents developed upon filing:

- The citation (also called the notice)

- The inventory

Documents developed in preparation for the hearing before the Court:

- Medical Certificate

- Affidavit and Treatment Plan

- Report of Guardian ad Litem

- Proposed Findings on Substituted Judgement

- Motion to Excuse Ward for attendance

- Decree of Permanent Guardianship

- Motion for Approval of Fees

- Statement of Services to be Provided by Guardian

- Order for Allowance of Guardian's Expenses

---

[26] In rare cases where the proposed ward has not been medically evaluated, the petitioner may request that the court order an evaluation, and in an emergency, appoint a temporary guardian, pending the evaluation.

Documents developed after the Guardian's appointment:

- Annual accounts

- Letter to Medicaid

- Petition to Terminate Guardianship

The Petition (Appendix 6-A)

The petition form can be obtained from the Register's office of the **Probate Court**. When a prospective guardian visits the court, he or she should obtain copies of all the forms required (the medical certificate and the bond form) and inquire about the filing fee (in 2003, $95.00) or, in the alternative, request an Affidavit of Indigency form. Massachusetts law (G.L. c. 261 § 27) provides access to the courts for indigents and low-income persons by requiring the court to waive filing fees and other costs where the party meets the indigency standards, that is, can show an inability to pay such court-related costs. See the self explanatory Affidavit of Indigency in Appendix 6-B.

In filling out the petition, the petitioner informs the court of the relevant details of the proposed ward's situation and describes the order or decree which the petitioner is seeking.

Identify the county in which the proposed ward resides. Leave the Docket Number blank, since that number will be assigned by the Court when the petition is filed.

Check which box describes the proposed ward. Check *Mental illness* if the medical certificate indicates that the proposed ward does indeed suffer from a mental illness or a suspected mental illness. A proposed ward in a coma is not mentally ill, but rather may be incapacitated by a physical illness (inability to communicate), in which case the third box should be checked. Where the proposed ward is an elderly nursing home resident, the medical certificate may describe a dementia that results from symptoms of a physical nature, like Alzheimer's or Parkinson's disease, and a physician may be unwilling to indicate a mental illness.

Very few nursing home residents are mentally retarded, and if the proposed ward is such a person, that is, developmentally disabled, there is a significantly different guardianship process, where the medical certificate is completed by a team of experts. Consult with the local ARC (Association for Retarded Citizens) or the Massachusetts Department of Mental Retardation for assistance.

The *Special Request* section requires that the petitioner(s) inform the court if the authority being requested is to: 1. authorize treatment of the ward with anti-psychotic medications in accordance with a treatment plan (*Rogers*) (see Appendix 6-A-2 for a list of the anti-psychotic medications generally in use in 2004), or 2. authorize the ward's admission or commitment to a mental health or mental retardation facility (Technically, the law does not require that the guardian obtain specific authority to admit the proposed ward to a nursing home, but the petitioners are well advised to make it clear if such authority is being sought), or 3. authorize or refuse extraordinary medical treatment (e.g., life supports such as feeding tubes or artificial respiration, amputation, or kidney dialysis.) If any of these boxes are checked, the court will appoint an attorney to represent the ward and may appoint a guardian *ad litem* to investigate the facts of the case and report back to the court.

The petitioners must be identified and must check which box describes their status or standing to file the petition.

The proposed ward must be identified by name and home address. If the ward is a nursing home resident, the home address is filled in here. If the nursing home resident has been in the facility for so long that there is no longer any home address, then the nursing home address may be used. The petitioner next checks the box corresponding to the box checked at the top of the petition form, regarding whether the proposed ward is mentally ill, developmentally disabled, or physically incapacitated and unable to communicate.

All of the apparent or presumptive heirs of the ward must be listed by name, address, and relationship. Heirs are persons who are legally entitled to share in the estate of a deceased person. If a person dies with a valid will in effect (**testate**), the beneficiaries named in the will are the heirs. If a person dies without a will in effect (**intestate**), then a Massachusetts statute (G.L. c. 190 § 1; see Appendix 6-A-1 for a summary) prescribes what blood relatives share in the estate. The petitioner should list all such heirs, including the beneficiaries of any will of which the petitioners are aware. If the heirs are too numerous to list on the petition, enter *See attached list*, and attach a complete list of all heirs. Heirs must be given notice of the proceedings and have the right to intervene.

A veteran or the spouse or widow/er of a veteran may be eligible for benefits from the federal Department of Veterans Affairs. If there is some doubt, contact the Fiduciary Unit of the **VA** for assistance.

On the back of the form, nominate the person(s) or entity(ies) to be appointed the guardian(s), and identify any specific authority to be conferred on the guardian by the court. The form also indicates that an agency, such as a non-profit organization with expertise in providing guardianship services, may be appointed guardian rather than a person or persons.

If any of the heirs at law wish to assent to the petition, there is space for them to do so; such assents bolster the standing of the petitioners and may obviate the need for giving notices to such heirs later on in the proceedings.

The petition must be signed by the petitioners under the penalties of perjury. If the petitioners are not represented by counsel, they are *pro se*, that is, representing themselves and must be identified in the space following *For Petitioners*. If the proposed ward is represented by counsel, identify that attorney under *For Respondent*. Otherwise, leave the space blank.

The space headed *PETITION-DECREE* is filled in by court officials.

The Medical Certificate (Appendix 6-C)

The Medical Certificate—Guardianship must be filled out and signed by a physician who has examined the proposed ward/patient within 30 days of the filing of the petition, and later, within 30 days of any request for action by the court. In guardianship proceedings, the judge will always insist on current information regarding the proposed ward's medical condition. The treating or examining physician should be familiar with this form and should give the court specific information about the patient's condition, diagnosis and symptoms, prescribed treatment, and the necessity for the appointment of a guardian because of the patient's limitations. For a patient in a hospital or a resident of a nursing home, the petitioner should have no difficulty obtaining a medical certificate since any treating physician understands that informed consent is required for all medical care being furnished to a patient.

The Bond (Appendix 6-D)

Along with the petition, the medical certificate, and the filing fee (or Affidavit of Indigency), the petitioners must also submit a Bond form to the court. The judge will not appoint the guardian without first approving a fiduciary bond to ensure that the proposed ward's resources are protected against the misconduct of a dishonest guardian.

In the space under which appears, *type of fiduciary*, enter the appropriate title, either *Temporary Guardian* or *Permanent Guardian*. The bond will be either without **sureties**, with personal sureties, or with corporate sureties:

Without Surety: The judge will rarely allow a bond without sureties, but may do so when the guardian is appointed as the guardian of the person and not the estate of the ward. A guardian of the person has no authority relative to the ward's income or assets, and presumably the court need not be concerned about such a guardian's bond when the financial affairs of the ward are not involved.

With Personal Surety: The court requires that two persons sign as guarantors of the integrity of the guardian and in essence represent to the court that they will insure the fiduciary's honesty and trustworthiness in carrying out the duties of guardian. The sureties must understand that they are genuinely insurers, and can be sued on the bond if the guardian is found to have misappropriated the ward's finances. When the proposed ward has significant assets, the court may inquire about the financial ability of the sureties to meet their obligations.

With Corporate Sureties: Where the ward has substantial or significant assets or income or the court concludes that personal sureties do not afford sufficient protection of the ward's finances, a corporate surety will be required. In such a case, the prospective guardian must obtain a corporate bond from an insurance company that issues such coverage for fiduciaries.

Identify the name of the estate, that is, the proposed ward and the name and address of the prospective guardian/fiduciary. (The term "fiduciary" appears because this form is used in other Probate Court contexts, for example in the appointment of an executor of an estate, etc.)

The bond form calls for the estimated value of any real estate in which the proposed ward has any interest. A guardian must obtain the permission of the court before taking any action affecting the ward's ownership of real estate. If a guardian plans to sell, transfer, or mortgage the ward's real estate, the guardian must ask the court for license to do so.

The estimated personal estate of the proposed ward must also be entered in the space provided. The personal estate consists of anything owned by the proposed ward that is not real estate. The bond is approved on the strength of the petitioners' estimation of the estate, but, once appointed, if the guardian discovers that the assets were substantially underestimated, a revised and more accurate bond must be filed.

The Penal Sum of the Bond requires the calculation of 150% of the estimated personal estate of the proposed ward. Any value of real estate is not part of the equation because the court supervises that aspect of the ward's holdings through the licensure process. If Agatha Adams has $1,800.00 in the bank, the penal sum is 150% of that value or $2,700.00.

The prospective guardian/fiduciary and the two personal sureties sign at the appropriate spaces. As explained on the reverse side of the bond form, a surety must be a resident of Massachusetts. If a corporate surety is used, the insurance company will endorse the bond in the space provided.

At the very bottom of the bond, the judge approves the bond as the last step before appointing the guardian by decree.

Motion for Appointment of Temporary Guardian (Appendix 6-E)

Once the petition is filed, the normal course is for the court to issue a citation or notice to be served on all interested parties (see Appendix 6- J). The petitioners serve the notices as prescribed by the court, either in hand or by mailing or publication in a designated newspaper's legal notice section. The notice contains a "return day," that is, a date by which any person objecting to the petition must file a written appearance on or before 10:00 a.m. on the return day. If no objections are filed and the papers are otherwise in order with no further review or actions to be taken by the court, the guardian will receive a copy of the decree of appointment.

Where there is an urgent need for the appointment of a guardian, however, and the emergency attention of the court is required to make such an appointment promptly, the petitioners may file a motion for the appointment of a temporary guardian. A temporary guardian is appointed by the court for a 90-day period, but only when the petitioner shows that there is an emergency, that there is a risk of a particular harm to the proposed ward that the petitioner seeks to avoid, and that the actions requested of the court by the petitioners are reasonably necessary to avoid that harm. The motion must be accompanied by an affidavit or affidavits sufficiently in support of the motion to convince the court to grant the relief sought.

Affidavit for Temporary Guardianship (Appendix 6-F)

The affidavit or affidavits must allege under the penalties of perjury the nature of the emergency, the harm to be avoided, and the reasonableness of the action requested of the court to avoid the harm. Need for emergency surgery is a typical basis for the appointment of a temporary guardian and requires affidavits from the petitioner and the treating physician and/or surgeon.

Motion to Appoint Counsel for Ward (Appendix 6-G)

In Rogers and Brophy guardianships, the court must appoint counsel for the proposed ward, and generally speaking, the court will pay the fees of the counsel appointed. Depending on the nature of the case, the court may pay other costs as well, for example, the costs of a medical expert witness. The court has authority to appoint counsel for the ward in every case but generally does so only when there is an obvious need, such as when the ward objects to the proceedings.

Physician's Affidavit and Treatment Plan (Appendix 6-H)

Where the medical treatment plan for the ward involves the administration of anti-psychotic medications, the physician's affidavit and treatment plan must also be submitted to the court.

Draft (or Proposed) Findings of Fact and Conclusions of Law (Appendix 6-I)

The court may require that the petitioner submit proposed findings of fact and conclusions of law at the time of appointment of either the temporary or permanent guardian. This document can speed the process, because the petitioners, who have knowledge of the ward's circumstances can, in effect, summarize the facts for the court to review and approve. Proposed findings of fact are a list of the important facts about the ward, and the court will agree to adopt the proposed facts as long as the petitioners have submitted testimony or documentary evidence to support the facts. Proposed conclusions of law recite the law, that is, the statutes, court decisions, or other authorities that apply to the facts of the case.

Citation or Notice (Appendix 6-J)

After the petition is filed, the court issues a citation that explains how the notice of the petition is to be given to all parties of interest. The petitioner must return the citation and certify that the citation has been complied with.

Temporary Decree of Guardianship (Appendix 6-K)

If all goes well, the court will appoint a temporary guardian as requested by the petitioners. Again, to expedite the process, the petitioners should come to court with a completed decree form, ready to be signed by the judge. The temporary guardianship is for only 90 days, but the court may extend the term of the temporary guardianship if for some reason the permanent guardianship cannot be granted by the expiration date of the temporary guardianship.

Permanent Decree of Guardianship (Appendix 6-L)

At the end of the process, a permanent guardian will be appointed.

Inventory (Appendix 6-M)

Upon appointment of a guardian, whether temporary or permanent, the court issues an inventory form on which the guardian is required to list the assets of the ward. The inventory must be completed and filed with the court within 90 days. The inventory is important and will be the basis for the future accounts that the guardian must file annually with the court.

Motion for Allowance of Guardianship Costs/fees (Appendix 6-N)

For a *Rudow* guardian to be compensated for his or her services to the ward, the petitioner must submit a motion for the allowance of costs and fees. The motion should explain the work done by the guardian, and an affidavit should be submitted to support the claim. The *Rudow* regulations are found in Appendix 6-O.

Model Letter to Medicaid (Appendix 6-P)

Once a guardian has been appointed, the procedure to be followed to implement the *Rudow* mechanism for payment is to submit a letter to Medicaid, along with copies of the decree of appointment, and the order of the Probate Court that approved the fees and costs. The guardian is compensated when the Medicaid program revises the ward's PPA for the next 12- month period; one-twelfth of the fees/costs are recovered each month. Thereafter, the guardian must file an affidavit annually with Medicaid that conforms with the requirements of the *Rudow* regulations at 130 C.M.R. § 520.126(E)(3)(d). See Appendix 6-O. The affidavit must describe the guardianship services provided and must include the assertion that the guardian has attended and participated in the quarterly care plan meetings held for the resident at the nursing home.

Accounts (Appendix 6-Q)

Each year the guardian must submit an annual account by which the guardian informs the court of the state of the ward's assets, income, and expenses. The account describes the period covered, and accounts for assets and income (Schedule A), expenses (Schedule B) and the remaining balance of the ward's estate (Schedule C).

Petition to Discharge Guardianship (Appendix 6-R)

If the ward recovers and is no longer incapacitated, there is a procedure for discharging the guardian or terminating the guardianship. For example, suppose that medical tests find an operable tumor as the suspected source of Agatha Adams' dementia, and surgery succeeds in restoring her to sound mental health. Where the medical certificate attests to her recovery and regained capacity, this petition asks to have the guardianship terminated.

Appendices to Chapter 6

6-A   Petition

6-A1   Law of Intestate Succession (Identifying Heirs at Law)

6-A2   Current List of Anti-psychotic Medications in Use

6-B   Affidavit of Indigency

6-C   Medical Certificate

6-D   Bond

6-E   Motion for Appointment of Temporary Guardian

6-F   Affidavit for Temporary Guardian

6-G   Motion to Appoint Counsel for the Ward

6-H   Physician's Affidavit and Treatment Plan

6-I   Draft Findings of Fact and Conclusions of Law

6-J   Citation/Notice

6-K   Temporary Decree of Guardianship

6-L   Permanent Decree of Guardianship

6-M   Inventory

6-N   Motion for Allowance of Fees/costs

6-O   "Rudow" Regulations

6-P   Model Letter to Medicaid

6-Q   Guardian's Account

6-R   Petition to Discharge Guardianship

6-A

NORFOLK Division

Commonwealth of Massachusetts
The Trial Court
Probate and Family Court Department

Docket No. _____

GUARDIANSHIP PETITION
GUARDIAN OF PERSON - AND ESTATE
Name of proposed ward __AGATHA T. ADAMS__

Please check applicable box and/or strike out inapplicable language where appropriate.
Basis for the Guardianship:

☒ *Mental Illness*   ☐ *Mental Retardation*   ☐ *Physical Incapacity or Illness*

Special Requests:

☒ for court authorization to treat with antipsychotic medication(s) in accordance with the treatment plan

☐ for court authorization to admit or commit to a mental health or mental retardation facility

☐ extraordinary medical authority

To the Justices of the Probate and Family Court:
RESPECTFULLY represents

PETITIONER (1)

__REBECCA THATCHER__
(PRINT name of petitioner)

PETITIONER (2)

__MELBA MAZOLA__
(PRINT name of petitioner)

that they are - he/she is:

☐ parent(s)

☒ two (or more) relatives or friends

☐ a nonprofit corporation organized under the laws of the Commonwealth

☐ an agency within the Executive Office of Human Services or Educational Affairs.

AND that _____ __AGATHA T. ADAMS__ _____ whose address is
(name of proposed ward)

__7 CARMODY COURT__ __QUINCY__ __NORFOLK__ __MA__ __02171__
(street address) (city or town) (county) (state) (zip code)

☒ is incapable of taking care of himself/herself by reason of mental illness.

☐ is mentally retarded to the degree that he/she is incapable of making informed decisions with respect to the conduct of his/her personal and/or financial affairs.

☐ is unable to make or communicate informed decisions due to physical incapacity or illness.

List **all** heirs apparent or presumptive of ward:

NAME (Please indicate if person is a minor or incompetent)	RESIDENCE	RELATIONSHIP
REBECCA THATCHER	10 DOWNING ST., GREAT BARRINGTON MA 02130	NIECE
MELBA MAZOLA	100 EASTERN ST., SALEM MA 01970	NIECE
URIAH CONTI	1 SARATOGA ST., BELMONT MA 02478	NEPHEW

The ward ☒- is not - entitled to benefits, estate, or income paid or payable through the United States Veterans Administration.

[Guardianship of mentally retarded persons ONLY]

☐ A Clinical Team report is filed with this petition. (See, G.L.M. c. 201, §6A and Uniform Probate Court Practice XXIX(A))

CJ-P 110 (10/97)

fcpfc - c.g.f.

(GUARDIANSHIP PETITION BACK)

WHEREFORE, the petitioner(s) pray(s) that _REBECCA THATCHER_
(name of proposed guardian(l))

10 DOWNING ST. GREAT BARRINGTON _MA_ _02130_
(street address) (city or town) (state) (zip code)

- and _____
(name of proposed guardian(2), if applicable)

_____
(street address) (city or town) (state) (zip code)

— or some other suitable person - be appointed the guardian of the person - and - the estate of the ward.

FURTHERMORE the petitioner(s) request(s):

☒ court authorization to treat with antipsychotic medication(s) in accordance with the treatment plan.

☐ court authorization to admit or commit to a mental health or mental retardation facility.

☐ court authorization for the following extraordinary medical procedure(s): _____

The Petitioner(s) certify(ies) under the penalties of perjury that - the ward's estate does not exceed $100.00 and that - the statements contained herein are true to the best of his/her/their knowledge and belief.

Dated: _JUNE 10, 2003_

PETITIONER (1) _Rebecca Thatcher_
(signature of petitioner)

10 DOWNING ST.
(street address)

GREAT BARRINGTON MA 02130
(city or town) (state) (zip code)

Tel. No. (_123_) _456 - 7890_

PETITIONER (2) _Nella Nazola_
(signature of petitioner)

100 EASTERN ST.
(street address)

SALEM MA 01970
(city or town) (state) (zip code)

Tel. No. (_231_) _456 - 7809_

The undersigned hereby assent(s) to the foregoing petition.

Nella Nazola

PETITION - DECREE

Filed: _____
Citation issued: _____
Returnable: _____
Allowed: _____

For Petitioner(s):

REBECCA THATCHER PRO SE
(name)

10 DOWNING ST.
(street address)

GREAT BARRINGTON MA 02130
(city or town) (state) (zip code)

Tel. No. (_123_) _456-7890_

B.B.O. # _X_

For Respondent:

_____
(name)

_____
(street address)

_____
(city or town) (state) (zip code)

Tel. No. ( ) _____

B.B.O. # _____

INSTRUCTIONS

1. Refer to G.L.M. c. 201, §§ 6, 6A,6B, 7; Probate Court Rule 2913; and, Uniform Probate Practice XXII and XXII(A).
2. A bond must be furnished.
3. If certified that the ward's estate is less than $100.00, no filing fee is required. If the ward's estate is $100.00 of more, a $50.00 filing fee, a $30.00 bond and $10.00 surcharge must be paid upon filing.
4. A Medical Certificate must be filed in accordance with Uniform Probate Practice XXII.

6-A1

MASSACHUSETTS LAW OF DESCENT AND DISTRIBUTION
LAW OF INTESTATE SUCCESSION (G.L. c. 190 S 1)

This chart demonstrates how your estate is divided or distributed in the event that you die intestate, that is, without a will:

IF YOU ARE SURVIVED BY:	YOUR ESTATE IS DISTRIBUTED:
1. Spouse and child/ren	One half to spouse One half to children
2. Spouse, no children, but next of kin (including parents, siblings, niece, nephew, aunt, uncle, cousin, etc.)	Where the estate is less than $200,000, all to spouse. If the estate is larger than $200,000, the first $200,000 plus one-half of everything in excess of $200,000 to spouse. The remainder to next of kin in this order: Parent(s), siblings, nieces and nephews, grandparents, uncles and aunts, cousins.
3. Spouse, no child, no next of kin	All to spouse
4. No spouse, one or more children	All to children
5. No spouse, no child, but next of kin	All to next of kin, in the order described above in 2.
6. No spouse, no child, no next of kin	All "escheats" to the Commonwealth of Mass., that is, all is turned over to the State, because there are no heirs or beneficiaries.

6-A2

ANTIPSYCHOTIC MEDICATIONS

Typical Antipsychotics

Brand name	Generic name	Usual daily dose (mg.)	Routes of administration
Haldol	Haloperidol	2-80	Oral
Haldol decanoate	Haloperidol decanoate	50-200	IM
Prolixin	Fluphenazine HCI	up to 20	Oral
Prolixin decanoate	Fluphenazine decanoate	2.5-50	IM
Orap	Pimazide	2-20	Oral
Stelazine	Trifluoperazine	up to 40	Oral
Trilafon	Perphenazine	12-64	Oral
Navane	Thiothixene	15-60	Oral
Serentil	Mesoridazine	75-400	Oral
Loxitane	Loxapine	60-100	Oral
Moban	Molindone	50-200	Oral
Mellaril	Thioridazine	up to 400	Oral
Thorazine	Chlorpromazine	75-900	Oral

Atypical Antipsychotics

Brand name	Generic name	Usual daily dose (mg)	Routes of administration
Clozaril	Clozapine	250-900	Oral
Risperdal	Risperidone	0.5-8	Oral
Zyprexa	Olanzapine	10-30	Oral
Seroquel	Quetiapine	50-750	Oral

Experimental Antipsychotics

Brand name	Generic name	Usual daily dose (mg)	Routes of administration
Zoldex	Ziprasidone	20-80	Oral
Unknown	Aripiprazole	5-30	Oral
Zomaril	Iloperidone	6-20	Oral

Antidepressants

Brand name	Generic name	Usual daily dose (mg)	Routes of administration
Elavil	Amitriptylline	50-150	Oral
Norpramin	Desipramine	100-200	Oral
Tofranil	Imipramine	75-200	Oral
Sinequan	Doxepin	75-150	Oral
Asendin	Amoxapine	200-400	Oral
Vivactil	Protiptyline	40-60	Oral
Desyrel	Trazodone	150-400	Oral
Nardil	Phenelzine	15-90	Oral
Parnate	Tranylcypromine	30	Oral
Prozac	Fluoxetine	20-80	Oral
Zoloft	Sertraline	50-200	Oral
Paxil	Paroxetine	20-60	Oral
Celexa	Citalopram	10-30	Oral
Luvox	Fluvoxamine	100-300	Oral
Effexor, Effexor SR	Venlexafine	75-225	Oral
Serzone	Nefazodone	300-600	Oral
Wellbutrin	Bupropion	300	Oral
Remeron	Mirtazapine	7.5-4.5	Oral
Vestra	*Reboxetine*	*Not yet determined*	*Oral*

Mood Stabilizers

Brand name	Generic name	Usual daily dose (mg)	Routes of administration
Lithane, Eskalith	Lithium	400-2400	Oral
Depakote	Divalproex sodium	750-2500	Oral
Tegretol	Carbamazepine	300-1600	Oral
Klonopin	Clonazepam	2-6	Oral
Lamictal	Lamotrizine	300-500	Oral
Neurontin	Gabapentin	900-3600	Oral

**The author acknowledges the contributions of
Rose M. Cain, Esq., Elder quest, P.C., Natick, MA 01760**

6-B

INSTRUCTIONS FOR USERS OF AFFIDAVIT OF INDIGENCY
AND ITS SUPPLEMENT

A state statute provides that if you cannot pay for court fees or costs, you may be able to have the state pay for them. These instructions describe who is eligible and how to use this law.

Who Is Eligible? - You are eligible for a waiver, substitution or state payment of fees and costs if any one of the following applies to you:

Category (A) You receive public assistance under one of the following programs: Massachusetts Transitional Aid to Families With Dependent Children; Massachusetts Emergency Aid to Elderly, Disabled & Children; Federal Supplemental Security Income; Massachusetts MassHealth (formerly Medicaid) or Massachusetts Veterans Benefits; or

Category (B) Your income, after taxes, does not exceed 125% of the current Federal Poverty Line. This Poverty Line is revised annually, and the current chart should be posted in your local courthouse. If you do not find it there, please ask the Clerk's office where it is or for a copy; or

Category (C) You cannot pay the court fees or costs without depriving yourself or those who are dependent on you of the necessities of life, including food, shelter and clothing.

If you are *currently* confined in prison or jail and do not seek your immediate release but are suing a "state or county agency, official or employee" about something "arising out of or resulting from a condition of or occurrence during confinement," *and* you are seeking court payment of "normal" costs (see definition below), please get from the Clerk's office separate forms for prisoners which you must complete in order to qualify for a waiver. You can use the general forms for non-prisoners if you are asking the court to pay for "extra" fees. Regardless of which forms you use you might find the information below useful.

What Fees And Costs are Covered? - All fees and costs (other than attorneys fees) involved in the prosecution or defense of "any civil, criminal or juvenile proceeding or appeal in any court" are eligible for waiver, substitution or payment by the Commonwealth. When you prepare your application, please identify those costs which you need waived or paid for the initial or next steps of your court case. For example, if you are filing a case in court and you need a waiver of the court filing fee, prepare an application for waiver of that fee. If, in addition, you need to have a sheriff or other officer serve court process, or you need publication of notice, include your estimates of these costs also. If, at a later time, you need waiver or payment of other court costs (such as costs for subpoenas of witnesses to hearings, costs of taking depositions of witnesses, etc.) you should make a separate application at that time.

The fees and costs which can be waived or paid by the state are divided into two categories:

(1) **Normal fees and costs** are those that "a party normally is required to pay in order to prosecute or defend the particular type of proceeding." They include, for example:

- Court filing fees and surcharges, and also appeal fees and surcharges
- Other court fees for issuing or certifying papers or for photocopies.
- Constable or sheriff fees for serving court process, witness subpoenas, or other court papers.

• Costs of publishing notices relating to a court action.

If you are requesting only normal fees and costs, and your affidavit appears regular and complete on its face and indicates that you are indigent, the Clerk will allow your request immediately "without hearing and without the necessity of appearance of any party or counsel." The Clerk will waive the fees or costs completely, order them to be paid by the Commonwealth, or substitute "an alternative means at lower or no cost [that] is substantially equivalent and . . . does not materially impair the rights of any party." If your affidavit is not regular and complete or you do not appear to be indigent, the clerk-magistrate will promptly present your request to a Judge for decision within 5 days. The Judge will either grant your request without a hearing or you will be notified of a hearing date.

If you are a prisoner, a Judge will need to act on your application after first ordering the facility where you are confined to produce a copy of your canteen account for the last six months. You may ask the court to order payment of the cost of serving the summons and complaint in the meantime, however, so your case can begin.

(2)   **Extra fees and costs** are those that are "in addition to those a party is normally required to pay in order to prosecute or defend [the] case, which result when a party employs or responds to a procedure not necessarily required in the particular type of proceeding." They include, for example:

• Costs of expert testing, examination or testimony
• Cassette copies for indigent parties not represented by a public defender
• Appeal bonds

If you are requesting any extra fees and costs, the Clerk will promptly present your request to a Judge for decision within 5 days. The Judge may allow your request without a hearing, but will not deny your request without holding a hearing. In reviewing a request for extra fees or costs, the Judge will decide whether the document, service or object is reasonably necessary to assure you as effective a prosecution, defense or appeal as you would have if you were financially able to pay.

"Normal" and "extra" fees and costs do not include attorneys' fees.

How Do I Apply? - You should complete the Affidavit of Indigency form that applies to you. If you claim eligibility under Category (C) above, you must also complete the Supplement to Affidavit of Indigency form. File your papers with the Clerk of the court where your case has been filed (or where you are seeking to file it). Court Clerks must accept your initial court papers when you present them, even if you have not then obtained a waiver of the filing fee. If the fee is later waived, the date of filing your court papers will be the day you first presented them to the Clerk.

What is the Federal Poverty Line? - If you want to qualify under Category (B) above (income, after taxes, which is less than 125% of the Federal Poverty Line), you should consult a chart of these income limits which should be posted in your local courthouse. If you cannot find this chart, go to the Clerk's office and find out where it is or ask to be given or to read a copy. This Poverty Line is increased every year in February or March, and so the court should have an up-to-date schedule.

How Do I Estimate the Costs? - There are places on the form where you can give the cost (if you know it) or give your best estimate of the cost of the particular fee or service that you need. If you do not know what the cost will be, give your best description of what you need. The court should approve your application, if you are otherwise eligible, even though you have not filled in complete information about the costs.

What Are the Situations in Which I Can Get a Substitution of a Service? - Under the law, a court can order that a different (or substitute) method of performing a certain act or service be allowed, rather than a less convenient or more expensive one. For example, in some situations a court might order that notice of filing a court action be made by posting in certain locations rather than by publishing the notice in a newspaper. In oth situations you may be able to take depositions using tape recorders rather than using a more expensive stenographer. If you have a request for a substitute method, please ask for it in your application. The court ma itself, order a less expensive or easier substitution. However, the judge may order you to pay a partial fee or co rather than to waive it if you are otherwise eligible for waiver or state payment.

If you are a prisoner bringing an action in Superior Court, you will receive a summons and be instructed to serv it with your complaint by certified mail. You can ask for permission to use regular mail if paying the cost of certified mail presents a hardship. If you are filing a case in another court, you can ask for permission to serve l certified or regular mail.

Can I Appeal A Denial? - Yes. If you disagree with any decision of the Clerk or Assistant Clerk, you can request a review by the judge. If you disagree with a decision of a Judge, you can appeal to the next court leve There are short deadlines for doing this, so you must act quickly. Consult the Clerk's office for information about how to do this.

Are the Indigent Court Costs Papers That I File in Court Confidential? - Yes, these papers are not available to the general public or to any other party in the case, but are only available to authorized court personnel and to you and your attorney or your other authorized representative. If you want an authorized representative other than your attorney to see or get copies of these documents, you should prepare a written consent so that a designated individual will have authority to do that. Any other party to the case, or their authorized representative, does not have access to these records unless that party gets a court order giving permission. Also, when you file an application or an appeal under the indigent court costs law, you are not required to give copies of any of these documents to any other party in the case.

INSTRUCTIONS TO COURTS ON THE ADMINISTRATION OF THE INDIGENT COURT COSTS LAW

Accompanying these Instructions are revised forms to be effective May 5, 2003 under the state's Indigent Court Costs Law, c.261, §§27A - G and 29. Please note that, for the first time, this court has included instructions to applicants as part of the Affidavit of Indigency forms. Previously, each Trial Court Department was authorized to draft its own instructions, if any. It is important to give the same information to users so that the forms and procedures will be more easily understood. Trial Court Departments can supplement or modify these Instructions, as appropriate to their particular Departments, so long as the changes are not inconsistent with these Instructions. If a court department does so, it should submit its changes to the Chief Justice of the Supreme Judicial Court for quick review before they go into effect.

These are some comments that we make on the Indigent Court Costs Statute and forms, in order to provide guidance to you in administering this law.

1) **Partial Fees May Be Permitted** - In the decision of Underwood v. Appeals Court, 427 Mass. 1012 (1998), this court decided that the statute authorizes the assessment of a partial fee as a substitute for complete waiver of the fee or state payment of the cost. The judge should exercise reasonable discretion, considering the totality of the applicant's economic circumstances, before ordering payment of a partial fee.

2) **Instructions on Use of Inmate Forms** - Included in the packet is a separate set of forms designed to meet requirements under recent amendments to the law pertaining to inmate filings. These forms are for use only when the applicant: (1) is currently confined in a correctional institution; (2) has brought suit against a state or county agency, official or employee (except for a petition for relief from restraint under G.L. c. 248, §1); and (3) seeks waiver of "normal" (as opposed to "extra") fees and costs. *See* G.L. c. 261, § 29. If any of these three criteria are not met, the applicant and court personnel should use the general forms.

The special inmate forms include an affidavit of indigency form that requires the prisoner to supply the specific information required by § 29(b). The form incorporates a preamble that notifies inmates of the particular consequences of intentionally filing an affidavit that is false or is designed to abuse the judicial process, as set forth in § 29(f). Once the action is filed, the court must, under § 29(a), order the custodial official to produce a printout of the plaintiff/inmate's institutional canteen and savings accounts within 30 days so that the inmate's resources can be assessed. The packet includes a form order to the Commissioner of Correction or county sheriff for this purpose. The court may tentatively approve an inmate's application to permit service of process while the order to the correctional administrator and further review is pending. § 29(e). If, upon review of the inmate's application and account information, the court determines that the inmate is indigent, it may waive fees entirely; require a one-time partial payment toward the fees and costs; or order an initial payment and subsequent installment payments. § 29(d). The form notice of waiver sets forth these options and notifies the prisoner of his/her obligation under § 29(d)(3) to forward the court's order to the appropriate custodial official. The form also permits the inmate to authorize the custodian to debit and send to the court the payments that are ordered.

3) Acceptance of Court Papers Accompanying Filing Fee Waiver Requests - Sometimes applicants for waiver of filing fees present papers on a day which is within a statute of limitation or other time deadline (such as an appeal from a state agency adjudicatory hearing decision). As the statute states (c.261, §27C(1)), all papers offered for filing must be dated and accepted when they are first presented, and must be processed without delay. This means that no papers may be rejected because the filer has not yet obtained waiver of the filing fee. Rather, if the filing fee is later waived, the date of filing is the date of the original presentation of the papers.

4) Duties of Clerk - The statute requires that applications for waiver or state payment of normal fees or costs under Categories A (recipients of certain means-tested public benefit programs) and B (income is below 125% of the federal poverty line) must be approved by the Clerk (or the Assistant Clerk) without delay so long as they are regular on their face and raise no significant question about whether the applicant is indigent. G. L. c. 261, 27C(2). Except in prisoner cases, such papers should not be referred to a judge for decision, nor should further information be requested if the papers are properly completed. Also, the Clerk should not require an applicant to complete the Supplement to the Affidavit of Indigency form unless he or she is applying under Category C.

Applications under Category C, which requires the applicant to complete a Supplement to Affidavit of Indigency, can frequently be decided at the Clerk's level, based upon the information submitted. But if there are serious questions about whether the applicant meets the Category C standard, the application should be referred to a judge for decision.

5) Confidentiality of Papers - All papers relating to requests under the Indigent Court Costs Law are confidential and not available to the public. The only exceptions are that they are available to authorized court personnel and to the applicant and the applicant's attorney. They are not available to any other party or their authorized representative without a specific court order. If an authorized representative (other than an attorney) for an applicant seeks to review or to obtain copies of any of these documents, that person should present a written consent by the applicant before access is permitted.

6) Appeals - G. L. c. 261, § 27C(3) provides that if the affidavit is not regular on its face or does not indicate the applicant is indigent, the clerk or register shall bring it to the attention of a judge. Any denial or other decision by a Judge can be appealed to an appellate court under the procedures provided for in the statutes or rules. G. L. c. 261, § 27D.

7) Posting of Federal Poverty Line Information - A chart showing 125% of the current federal standards of poverty for different sized families must be posted in each local court in a place where litigants are likely to see it. These standards are updated by the federal government each year in February or March, and so courts should be sure that they have a current schedule posted. Each year, shortly after the federal change, the Supreme Judicial Court staff mails out a copy of the new schedule. If the schedule is not posted in the courthouse, applicants who need to review it are instructed to ask for a copy at the Clerk's office.

8) Estimated Costs - Applicants are asked to give their best estimates of the costs of the services whose waiver or state payment they are requesting. If they do not know the cost, they are asked to provide a reasonable description of what they need. Most applicants will not know the actual costs of many of these services. Therefore, courts should approve otherwise appropriate applications for waiver or state payment and insert in the approval the actual or estimated amount of the fee or service, as it is known to the court.

Commonwealth of Massachusetts

AFFIDAVIT OF INDIGENCY

AND REQUEST FOR WAIVER, SUBSTITUTION
OR STATE PAYMENT OF FEES & COSTS

(Note: If you are currently confined in a prison or jail and are not seeking immediate release under G.L. c. 248 §1, but you are suing correctional staff and wish to request court payment of "normal" fees (for initial filing and service), do not use this form. Obtain separate forms from the clerk.)

Court	Case Name and Number (if known)

Name of applicant_____

Address_____
(Street and number)   (City or town)   (State and Zip)

SECTION 1: Under the provisions of General Laws, Chapter 261, Sections 27A-27G, I swear (or affirm) as follows: **I AM INDIGENT** in that *(check only one)*:

☐ (A) I receive public assistance under Transitional Aid to Families with Dependent Children (TAFDC), Emergency Aid to Elderly, Disabled or Children (EAEDC), Supplemental Security Income (SSI), Medicaid (MassHealth) or Massachusetts Veterans Benefits Programs; *(circle form of public assistance received)*; or

☐ (B) My income, less taxes deducted from my pay, is $_____ per week/month/year *(circle period that applies)*, for a household of _____ persons, consisting of myself and _____ dependents; which income is at or below the court system's poverty level; *(Note: The court system's poverty levels for households of various sizes must be posted in this courthouse. If you cannot find it, ask the clerk. The court system's poverty level is updated each year.)* [List any other available household income for the circled period on this line: _____) or

☐ (C) I am unable to pay the fees and costs of this proceeding, or I am unable to do so without depriving myself or my dependents of the necessities of life, including food, shelter and clothing.

IF YOU CHECKED (C), YOU MUST ALSO COMPLETE THE SUPPLEMENT TO THE AFFIDAVIT OF INDIGENCY.

SECTION 2: *(Note: In completing this form, please be as specific as possible as to fees and costs known at the time of filing this request. A supplementary request may be filed at a later time, if necessary.)*

I request that the following **NORMAL FEES AND COSTS** be waived (not charged) by the court, or paid by the state, or that the court order that a document, service or object be substituted at no cost (or a lower cost, paid for by the state): *(Check all that apply and, in any "$____" blank, indicate your best guess as to the cost, if known.)*

☐ Filing fee and any surcharge. $_____

☐ Filing fee and any surcharge for appeal. $_____

☐ Fees or costs for serving court summons, witness subpoenas or other court papers. $_____

☐ Other fees or costs of $_____ for *(specify):*_____

_____

☐ Substitution *(specify):*_____

_____

SECTION 3: I request that the following **EXTRA FEES AND COSTS** either be waived (not charged), substituted or paid for by the state:

☐ Cost, $_____, of expert services for testing, examination, testimony or other assistance *(specify):*

_____

☐ Cost, $_____, of taking and/or transcribing a deposition of *(specify name of person):*_____

☐ Cassette copies of tape recording of trial or other proceeding, needed to prepare appeal for applicant not represented by Committee for Public Counsel Services (CPCS-public defender).

☐ Appeal bond

☐ Cost, $_____, of preparing written transcript of trial or other proceeding

☐ Other fees and costs, $_____, for *(specify)*_____

_____

☐ Substitution *(specify)*_____

_____

Date signed	Signed under the penalties of perjury
	x_____

By order of the Supreme Judicial Court, all information in this affidavit is CONFIDENTIAL. Except by special order of a court, it shall not be disclosed to anyone other than authorized court personnel, the applicant, applicant's counsel or anyone authorized in writing by the applicant.

This form prescribed by the Chief Justice of the SJC pursuant to G.L. c. 261, § 27B. Promulgated March , 2003

Commonwealth of Massachusetts

SUPPLEMENT TO AFFIDAVIT OF INDIGENCY
AND REQUEST FOR WAIVER, SUBSTITUTION
OR STATE PAYMENT OF FEES & COSTS

(Note: If you checked (C) on the AFFIDAVIT OF INDIGENCY, you must complete this form.)

Court	Case Name and Number (if known)

Name of applicant_____

Address_____

(Street and number)	(City or town)	(State and Zip)

Under the provisions of General Laws, Chapter 261, Sections 27A-G, I swear or affirm as follows:

1.   PERSONAL INFORMATION

    (a)   Date of Birth:_____

    (b)   Highest Grade Attained in School:_____

    (c)   Special Training:_____

    (d)   List any physical or mental disabilities which you wish to reveal and which affect your earning capacity or living expenses:

_____

_____

    (e)   Number of Dependents:_____

2.   INCOME AFTER TAXES (monthly):

    (a)   If from employment, list your occupation and your employer's name and address:

_____

_____

    (b)   Source of income, if not from employment: _____

_____

    (c)   My gross annual income for the past twelve months was: $_____

(d)   Gross Income (monthly): $ _____

(e)   Taxes Deducted (monthly):

        Federal Tax $ _____

        State Tax $ _____

        Social Security $ _____

        Medicare $ _____

        Other Taxes (specify) $ _____

        Total Taxes Deducted $ _____

(f)   Total Income After Taxes (*subtract 2(e) from 2(d)*): $ _____

(g)   If any other member of your household is employed, list occupation and name and address of his/her employer and monthly income after taxes:_____

_____

NET INCOME (monthly):

(a)   Income After Taxes (from Line 2(f)): $ _____

(b)   Expenses (monthly):

Rent or Mortgage	$ _____	Uninsured Medical Expenses	$ _____
Food	$ _____	Child Care	$ _____
Electricity	$ _____	Education Expenses for Children	$ _____
Gas	$ _____	Child Support	$ _____
Oil	$ _____	Clothing	$ _____
Water	$ _____	Laundry/Cleaning	$ _____
Telephone	$ _____	Car Insurance	$ _____
Health Insurance	$ _____	Transportation Expenses	$ _____

        Other *(specify):* $ _____

_____

        Total Expenses $ _____

(c)   Income After Taxes Minus Expenses (monthly) *(subtract 3(b) from 3(a))*: $ _____

4. **ASSETS**

    (a)   Own home? _____ Market Value $ _____

            Balance owed $ _____

    (b)   Own Car? _____ Year & Make _____

            Market Value $ _____ Balance Owed $ _____

    (c)   Bank Accounts (specify type and balance) _____

            _____

    (d)   Other Property Including Real Estate (specify type and value)_____

            _____

5. **DEBTS**

    (a)   Specify: _____

            _____

6. **MISCELLANEOUS**

    (a)   Other facts which may be relevant to your ability to pay fees and costs?

            _____

            _____

Signed under the penalties of perjury:

            Signature: _____

            Type/Printed Name: _____

            Address: _____

            Date: _____

By order of the Supreme Judicial Court, all information in this affidavit is CONFIDENTIAL. Except by special order of a court, it shall not be disclosed to anyone other than authorized court personnel, the applicant, applicant's counsel or anyone authorized in writing by the applicant.

This form prescribed by the Chief Justice of the SJC pursuant to G.L. c. 261, § 27B. Promulgated March , 2003

6-C

Commonwealth of Massachusetts
The Trial Court

NORFOLK Division   Probate and Family Court Department   Docket No. _____

MEDICAL CERTIFICATE — GUARDIANSHIP

To the Honorable Justices of the Probate and Family Court:

The undersigned hereby certifies under the penalties of perjury that I am a registered physician and that I personally examined____AGATHA T. ADAMS____
(name of proposed ward)

7 CARMODY COURT _____ QUINCY _____ MA
(street address)   _(city or town)_   _(state)_

on ___JUNE 2, 2003___
(date of examination)

and in my opinion the proposed ward:

☒   is a mentally ill person to the degree that he/she is incapable of caring for his/her personal and/ or financial affairs.

☐   is a person who is unable to make or communicate informed decisions due to physical incapacity.

THIS SECTION MUST BE COMPLETED FOR A GUARDIANSHIP PETITION

Describe in detail the diagnosis leading to the aforementioned opinion (including the types of decisions which the proposed ward has sufficient mental ability to make):

MS. ADAMS SUFFERS FROM DEMENTIA WITH ANXIETY AND DELUSIONS (A DISORDER OF MEMORY, ORIENTATION, MOOD, THOUGHT AND PERCEPTION). SHE IS QUITE CONFUSED AND HALLUCINATES. SHE HAS NO INSIGHT OR APPRECIATION OF HER MULTIPLE MEDICAL AND PSYCHIATRIC PROBLEMS. SHE IS UNABLE TO UNDERSTAND THE RISKS AND THE BENEFITS OF PROPOSED TREATMENT (RISPERIDONE TO TREAT AGITATION AND DISTRESS). MS. ADAMS

(OVER)

CJ-P 112 (10/93)

(MEDICAL CERTIFICATE — GUARDIANSHIP BACK)

IS NOT ABLE TO MAKE INFORMED DECISIONS ABOUT HER TREATMENT, FINANCES, OR NURSING HOME PLACEMENT/ADMISSION.

Date _JUNE 2, 2003_

_____
(signature)
VINCENT PHIBES, M.D.
(PRINT name)
GENERAL HOSPITAL
(address, including zip code)
10 MAIN ST.
QUINCY, MA 02171

Tel. No. (987) 654-3210

Uniform Probate Court Practice XXII.
A physician's certificate, when accepted, must be **dated** and the **examination** must have taken place within **thirty (30) days** prior to the entry of each decree, temporary or permanent.

6-D

Commonwealth of Massachusetts
The Trial Court
Probate and Family Court Department

NORFOLK **Division**   Docket No. _____

( ) **without**

Bond of _TEMPORARY GUARDIAN_ (X) **with Personal Surety**
(type of fiduciary)

( ) **with Corporate Surety**

Name of Estate _____AGATHA T. ADAMS_____ MA 02130

Name and Address of Fiduciary _REBECCA THATCHER, 10 DOWNING ST., GREAT BARRINGTON_

Estimated Real Estate _____0_____   Estimated Personal Estate _$1,800.00_

Penal Sum of Bond, (if applicable) _____$2,700.00_____

1, We, the undersigned fiduciary accept appointment as _TEMPORARY GUARDIAN_
and stand bound - in the aforesaid penal sum - with the undersigned surety or sureties - (if applicable) to perform the statutory conditions of said bond and declare the above estimate to be to my - our best knowledge and
belief.

Date _JUNE 10, 2003_ _____ _Rebecca Thatcher_
Signature of Fiduciary - Principal

(complete below only if this is a bond with personal sureties)

We, the undersigned, as sureties, stand bound jointly and severally in the aforesaid penal sum to perform the
statutory condition.

Personal Surety's Name and Address _MELBA MAZOLA 100 EASTERN AVE., SALEM_
_MA 01970_

Signature ___Melba Mazola___

Personal Surety's Name and Address _F. GERARD COUGHLIN, 290 WEST_
SIXTH ST., SOUTH BOSTON MA 02127

Signature ___F. G. Coughlin___

The above sureties are in my opinion sufficient.

_____   _____   _____
Signature   Office   City or Town

(complete below only if this is a Surety Company Bond)

We, the undersigned surety company, a corporation duly organized by law under the state of
_____ and having a usual place of business in _____

_____
(Massachusetts address)

stand bound as surety, in the aforesaid penal sum, to perform the statutory condition.

_____ by _____
Corporate Surety (name)   Signature and Title

_____, ss. _____, 20_____ examined and approved.

CJ-P 26 (j /89)

No.

_____

FIDUCIARY BOND

Filed _____ 19 . .

Approved _____ 19 _____

INSTRUCTIONS

Reference - Massachusetts General Laws Chapter 205, Section 1

This form covers the following fiduciaries:

Administrator - Administratrix

Public - cle bonis non — with the will annexed — de bonis with the will annexed

Executor - Executrix

Trustee under a will or written instrument

Temporary and permanent conservator, guaridan to minor, mentally ill or mentally retarded persons

Receiver of the property of an absentee

Sureties must be residents of Massachusetts or in the case of a Surety Company have a usual place of business in Massachusetts.

549

6-E

COMMONWEALTH OF MASSACHUSETTS
THE TRIAL COURT
PROBATE FAMILY COURT DEPARTMENT

NORFOLK COUNTY DIVISION   Docket No.

In Re: Guardianship of Agatha T. Adams

<u>MOTION FOR APPOINTMENT OF TEMPORARY GUARDIAN</u>

Now comes the petitioner, Rebecca Thatcher and moves that this Court appoint the said Rebecca Thatcher as the Temporary Guardian of Agatha T. Adams, to address the need for immediate and emergency action to deal with the proposed ward's medical treatment needs.

In support of this motion, the petitioner asserts that Agatha T. Adams, is currently a patient at the General Hospital in Quincy, and is in need of anti-psychotic medications to treat the anxiety and delusions she is experiencing as a result of her dementia. Her treating physician has prescribed Risperidone to treat the agitation and marked distress of the patient which had been interfering with the treatment of her physical ailments (rehabilitation for post fracture of left shoulder, congestive heart failure and chronic obstructive pulmonary disease). The proposed ward had a health care proxy, her sister Beatrice, who died on May 28, 2003. There is no one with authority to authorize the medical treatment needed or to affect a transfer of the proposed ward and admission to the Eveningtide Nursing Home in Quincy where there is currently a bed available and which is a more suitable environment for the proposed ward and the treatment needed.

The petitioners are the nieces of the proposed ward and are very familiar with her and can attest that she customarily followed her doctor's advice; her sister Beatrice was a retired nurse. Based on the petitioner's knowledge of the proposed ward's attitude toward medical care, Agatha would want to continue with the medical treatment prescribed and it is anticipated that she will adjust to the nursing home to the extent that her dementia permits.

WHEREFORE, the petitioner requests that the Court appoint Rebecca Thatcher as Temporary Guardian for a period of ninety days.

Respectfully submitted,

REBECCA THATCHER,

PRO SE PETITIONER,

Rebecca Thatcher

10 Downing Street

Great Barrington, MA 02130

Tel: (123) 456-7890

Date: June 10, 2003

6-F

Commonwealth of Massachusetts
The Trial Court
Probate and Family Court Department

NORFOLK **Division**   Docket No._____

AFFIDAVIT FOR TEMPORARY GUARDIANSHIP

Guardianship of ___AGATHA T. ADAMS___

I/We. __REBECCA THATCHER__ of __GREAT BARRINGTON, MA__
                    Print Name(s)

hereby state that:

1. On or about ___JUNE 10, 2003___, the situation of the proposed ward which
                              Date

requires emergency attention is THAT SHE NEEDS ANTI PYSCHOTIC MEDICATIONS
AND NEEDS TO BE ADMITTED TO THE EVENINGTIDE
NURSING HOME IN QUINCY WHERE THERE IS
CURRENTLY A BED AVAILABLE.

2. The petitioner(s) seek(s) to avoid the particular harm of: WITHOUT ANTI PSYCHOTIC
MEDICATION (RISPERIDONE), IT WILL IMPOSSIBLE TO
TREAT THE PATIENT DUE TO AGITATION AND ANXIETY
RELATED TO DEMENTIA; LOSS OF NURSING HOME BED
WILL EXTEND HOSPITAL STAY INDEFINITELY

3. The actions with regard to the proposed ward which are reasonably necessary to avoid the occurrence

of that harm are: A TEMPORARY GUARDIAN WILL HAVE LEGAL
AUTHORITY TO AUTHORIZE MEDICAL TREATMENT
AND SIGN ADMISSION PAPERS TO THE NURSING
HOME

4. Check one of the following: (NOT applicable to minors)

[X] The proposed ward has executed a Health Care Proxy and/or a Durable Power of Attorney (copy
attached) BUT THE AGENT IS DECEASED

[ ] The proposed ward has not executed a Health Care Proxy and/or a Durable Power of Attorney

[ ] I have been unable to determine if the proposed ward has executed a Health Care Proxy and/or
a Durable Power of Attorney

Signed this _10th_ day of _JUNE_ 20_03_, under the penalties of perjury.

Rebecca Thatcher
                              Signature(s)

CJ-P 113 (11/98)   pcpfc - c.g.f.

6-G

COMMONWEALTH OF MASSACHUSETTS
THE TRIAL COURT
PROBATE FAMILY COURT DEPARTMENT

NORFOLK COUNTY DIVISION   Docket No.

In Re: Guardianship of Agatha T. Adams

MOTION FOR APPOINTMENT OF COUNSEL

Now comes the petitioner Rebecca Thatcher and moves that this Court appoint legal counsel for Agatha T. Adams of Quincy. In support of this motion, the petitioner asserts that Agatha T. Adams has recently experienced a decline in her physical and mental condition. She is currently inpatient at the General Hospital in Quincy, where medical staff have recommended that the family initiate guardianship proceedings because she requires assistance with decision making, including the use and administration of antipsychotic medication, and the admission to a long term care facility. Given the above described circumstances, Agatha T. Adams should be independently represented by legal counsel during this process to assure that her rights are safeguarded and that medical decisions regarding the use of antipsychotic mediation will be in her best interest.

WHEREFORE, the petitioner requests that the Court appoint counsel.

_____

Rebecca Thatcher, Petitioner

Date:

6-H

COMMONWEALTH OF MASSACHUSETTS
THE TRIAL COURT
PROBATE FAMILY COURT DEPARTMENT

NORFOLK COUNTY DIVISION   Docket No.

In Re: Guardianship of Agatha T. Adams

<u>PHYSICIAN'S AFFIDAVIT</u>

I, Vincent Phibes, M.D., state to my best knowledge and belief that:

1. I am a registered physician with a specialty in psychiatry. I am a consulting psychiatrist for the Eveningtide Nursing Home and the Quincy Medical Center.

2. I have supervised and monitored the medication plan for Agatha Adams, since her admission to the hospital in May, 2003. I have had the opportunity to observe Ms. Adams periodically and to consult staff on medication changes.

BACKGROUND

3. Agatha Adams is an 88 year old woman who was admitted to the Quincy Medical Center in Quincy for a fractured shoulder in May, 2003. She no longer needs acute care, and has been evaluated and approved for admission to the Eveningtide Nursing Home in Milton. Prior to her admission, Ms. Adams lived alone in an elderly housing development; her sister, a retired nurse living in the same building, was her primary care giver. The sister died suddenly in May, and a niece, Becky Thatcher, found the patient lying injured in her apartment. Ms. Adams had been displaying symptoms of dementia, notably anxiety, agitation, and delusional thoughts prior to her admission but those symptoms have been elevated since her hospitalization. She has a prior history of congestive heart failure and chronic obstructive pulmonary disease. Ms. Adams has experienced over the past several years a progressive cognitive and functional decline consistent with Alzheimer's dementia. This is an irreversible, progressive brain illness that robs one of memory, orientation, ability to plan, organize and process information or execute tasks, and of the ability to reason.

4. These deficits have severely impaired Ms. Adams' insight and judgment. She has exhibited associated behavioral disturbances marked by anxiety, agitation and delusions. These symptoms have required the use of antipsychotic medication, Risperidone, to ease her agitation and distress. Risperidone continues to be helpful in the treatment of her psychotic symptoms.

5. Unfortunately, there is no chance of recovery, and Ms. Adams' prognosis is universally poor. Nonetheless, she may adjust to life at the nursing home and her family, her two nieces and some former neighbors, will visit her regularly.

TREATMENT PLAN

6. A Treatment Plan is attached.

RELIGIOUS BELIEFS

7. Ms. Adams has no known religious beliefs whose tenets prohibit the use of antipsychotic medications.

FAMILY SUPPORTS

8. Ms. Adams' family is supportive of the treatment plan and medication regimen recommended by the Quincy Medical Center and the Eveningtide Nursing Home.

MEDICATION

9. The following medication is recommended:

CONCLUSION

10. Ms. Adams is expected to make a good adjustment to the Eveningtide Nursing Home and the Risperidone is controlling the psychotic symptoms. Unfortunately, there is no chance of recovery but she can be cared for in safety and comfort with opportunities for social interaction and continued contact with her family and friends.

Signed under the penalty of perjury.

Date: _____

Vincent Phibes, M.D.

(Address)

COMMONWEALTH OF MASSACHUSETTS

NORFOLK, SS.

Probate and Family Court
Dept.Docket No.

_____

In Re:)

)

Guardianship of   )

_____   )

_____

AFFIDAVIT OF _____**, M.D.**

AS TO COMPETENCY AND PROPOSED TREATMENT PLAN FOR

_____

    I, _____, M.D., do hereby state to my best knowledge and belief:

1.   My name is _____, M.D. I am a registered physician and pyschiatrist employed by
_____.

2.   I supervise/consult on the treatment of _____ who is currently residing at _____.

3.   I have been supervising/consulting on the treatment of said patient since_____
_____.

4.   Since that date, I have had the opportunity to observe said patient in the following setting:

_____

_____

I have participated in case conferences and professional consultations concerning the patient. I have also reviewed the patient's medical records and am familiar with the patient's case history.

5.   I have conferred with the following clinical staff in rendering the opinion expressed in this affidavit:

_____

6.   The patient is a _____ year old _____ and is diagnosed with _____

_____. This disorder is characterized by the following symptoms or behaviors:

_____
_____

7.   Following is a brief personal history of the patient:

_____
_____
_____

8.   Following is the patient's history of treatment with antipsychotic medication:

   a) The patient has not been previously treated with antipsychotic medication. The patient was first treated in _____.

   b) Medications which have been used include the following:

   _____
   _____

   c) The effect on the use of these medications on the patient was as follows:_____

   d) The effect of the cessation of these medications on the patient was as follows:

   _____
   _____.

9.   (If applicable) The patient has experienced incidents or threats of dangerousness to self or others. These incidents include the following:

_____
_____
_____.

It is my opinion that adequate treatment of this patient requires the administration of antipsychotic medication as set forth it this affidavit.

It is my opinion that the patient is incompetent to make treatment decisions involving an antipsychotic medication.

10. The patient does not have the present ability to make informed decisions with respect to his/her personal affairs; specifically, he/she does not have the present capacity to make informed decisions regarding treatment with antipsychotic medication.

11. I based this conclusion on my observations and examinations of the patient and upon the following specific facts noted in the course of those observations and examinations:

(Circle applicable grounds for incompetency).

a) The patient does not understand the nature of his/her condition.

b) The patient does not understand the risks and benefits of the proposed plan of treatment.

c) The patient's mental retardation significantly impairs his/her judgment.

d) Other (state)

_____

_____

_____.

PROGNOSIS WITH TREATMENT

12. It is my opinion that prognosis with treatment is as follows:

_____

_____

_____.

PROGNOSIS WITHOUT TREATMENT

13. It is my opinion that if the below described treatment is not provided to this patient, then the prognosis is as follows:

_____

_____

_____.

PATIENT'S FAMILY

(Circle applicable statement)

14a.   The patient has no known family.

14b.   The patient has no family actively involved in the patient's treatment.

14c.   The patient's family has been supportive of the patient's treatment and has cooperated with facility staff.

14d.   Other (state):

_____

_____.

PATIENT'S EXPRESSED PREFERENCES REGARDING TREATMENT

15.   The patient is refusing/accepting antipsychotic medication. The patient's stated reasons for refusing/accepting medication are as follows:

_____

_____

_____.

RELIGIOUS BELIEFS AND IMPACT ON SUBSTITUTE JUDGMENT

16.   There is, to the best of my knowledge and belief, no evidence that the patient subscribes to any religious beliefs or convictions which would contribute to the patient's decisions regarding treatment as set forth in this affidavit.

PROBABILITY OF ADVERSE SIDE EFFECTS

17.   The name(s) of the proposed antipsychotic medication(s) is as follows:

_____

_____.

18.   The proposed medication may have the following side effects: sedation, dry mouth, dizziness, constipation, motor restlessness or tremors. These side effects are generally controllable with the use of anticholinergic medications such as Cogentin or Artane and disappear when antipsychotics are discontinued. A long term side effect of antipsychotics is Tardive Dyskinesia, an involuntary muscle movement disorder which generally affects the face, neck and mouth. The development of Tardive Dyskinesia is usually associ-

ated with long term care of high dose of the medications and generally occurs in 20% to 30% of the patients treated with the medications.

19. The patient's history of side effects to the proposed antipychotic medication, if any:_____.

20. The agents which will be used to counteract side effects, if any:

_____

_____.

TREATMENT PLAN

21. Treatment of choice:

a) Name of antipsychotic medication, dosage range (PO and IM):

_____

_____

b) Treatment duration:

_____

_____

22. Alternative antipsychotic medication(s):

a) Name of antipsychotic medication, dosage range (PO and IM):

_____

b) Treatment duration: _____

_____.

(13). Medication efficacy will be monitored in the following manner:

_____

_____

_____.

24. Effectiveness of the proposed treatment will be judged by the following criteria: (circle applicable criteria)

a) increased social activity

b) decrease in volatile affect and hostility

c) increased ability to plan

d) increased participation in work program and occupational therapy

e)   other (state): _____

25.   Long term planning for this patient includes the following:

_____

_____

_____.

SIGNED UNDER THE PAINS AND PENALTIES OF PERJURY THIS _____DAY OF _____, 2004.

_____

NAME

_____

ADDRESS

_____

_____

TELEPHONE

COMMONWEALTH OF MASSACHUSETTS

NORFOLK, SS.   Probate and Family Court
                                     Dept.Docket No.

```
                                  )
In Re:                            )
                                  )
Guardianship of                   )
_____                  )
```

PROPOSED ANTIPSYCHOTIC MEDICATION TREATMENT PLAN

In accordance with my affidavit dated _____, I recommend
the following antipsychotic medication treatment plan for _____:

1. ANTIPSYCHOTIC MEDICATION: _____, dosage range of

    _____ mg/day;

2. ALTERNATIVE ANTIPSYCHOTIC

    MEDICATION: _____, dosage range of

    _____mg/day;

3. ALTERNATIVE ANTIPSYCHOTIC

    MEDICATION: _____, dosage range of

    _____ mg/day.

SIGNED under the pains and penalty of perjury this_____day of_____, 2004.

_____

Signature

_____

Address

_____

_____

(___)_____

Telephone No.

6-I

COMMONWEALTH OF MASSACHUSETTS

ESSEX, SS

PROBATE AND FAMILY COURT
Docket No. 99- 1066—GI1

In Re: Guardianship of

Agatha Adams

FINDINGS OF FACT AND
CONCLUSIONS OF LAW

This case came before me for hearing on a motion for the appointment of a temporary guardian on October 25, 1999 and for appointment of permanent guardian on November 30, 1999, in both occasions after notice, hearing the parties, and examining their exhibits, I make the following Findings of Fact and Conclusions of Law:

1. This matter was brought before this Court on the petition of Nancy Drew, the niece of Agatha Adams, seeking authority to consent to medical treatment, for authority to monitor the administration of anti-psychotic medication and to admit the proposed ward to a nursing home. The attorney for the petitioner is Atticus Finch.

2. No counsel was appointed for the proposed ward, as it was represented to the court that there were no contested issues.

3. Agatha Adams did not attend either hearing.

4. The following documentary evidence was admitted into evidence: Medical Affidavit and Proposed Treatment Plan of John Kildare, M.D., dated October 21, 1999.

5. Dr. Kildare did not attend either hearing.

6. The respondent is 88 years of age and resides at 7 Carmody Court, Lynn, Massachusetts. Shewas admitted to the Gotham City Hospital on October 5, 1999, where she was diagnosed as having suffered a fractured left shoulder, with congestive heart failure, chronic obstructive pulmonary disease, and exhibiting dementia of some two years duration. She has been compliant with and has responded to therapies for her shoulder, but now needs long term care placement. She cannot be returned home, because her primary caregiver, a younger sister, died on October 4, 1999, at the age of 79.

Findings of Fact on Competence

1. The respondent is a mentally ill person who is not capable by reason of such mental illness of caring for herself and who does not have the present ability to make informed decisions regarding her medical treatment, including but not limited to treatment with anti-psychotic medications.

2. Specifically, the Court finds that the respondent is exhibiting dementia with delusions and depression, diagnosed as likely a combination of Alzheimer's disease and vascular dementia.

3. The Court has appointed the respondent's niece, Nancy Drew, as temporary guardian of the person and the estate of Agatha Adams on October 25, 1999. The Court finds her to be a suitable guardian. The Court finds that there is a need for substituted judgment on the matter of the guardian's request to give informed consent to medical treatment, including treatment with anti-psychotic medications.

FINDINGS OF FACT ON SUBSTITUTED JUDGMENT

1. The findings above on competency are not repeated but are considered here as applicable. In prior years, the respondent had made informed decisions for and against medical treatment, and in recent years she gave health care proxy authority to her sister, Beatrice, who was exercising that authority until she died on October 4, 1999. Due to the respondent's condition, she is not able to make such decisions.

2. The respondent has not expressed a preference which would inhibit compliance with the proposed treatment plan. Such representation is substituted by representation of the respondent's niece and acquaintances and that her religion and her own religious beliefs would not prevent her from accepting the proposed treatment.

3. The respondent has not expressed a preference for treatment by anti-psychotic medication and her niece and neighbors represent that the respondent has accepted treatment from doctors and medication in the past, prior to becoming mentally ill.

4. There would be no appreciable impact on the respondent's family should treatment be instituted or withheld other than the distress of her family should she require placement in a psychiatric facility.

5. The respondent's prognosis if treatment is not provided is that, in all likelihood, she will continue to deteriorate, will become unmanageable

and unsuitable for nursing home care and require commitment to a psychiatric facility. She will likely become markedly combative, paranoid, and will pose a danger to herself and others.

6.   The respondent's prognosis if treatment is provided is that she will enjoy relative stable health and will be well cared for in a nursing home, the least intrusive setting.

7.   The petition and treatment plan are offered in good faith and there is no conflict between the proposed treatment plan and the wishes of the family.

TREATMENT PLAN

A treatment plan, dated October 21, 1999, proposed by Dr. John Kildare, is attached hereto and incorporated by reference. The risks and benefits of the proposed treatment are set forth therein.

CONCLUSIONS OF LAW

I conclude, by a preponderance of the evidence that Agatha Adams is in need of anti-psychotic medications and of other medical treatment to which she is unable to give informed consent.

I conclude, beyond a reasonable doubt, after careful consideration of the evidence that, using a subjective test as to what Agatha Adams would do if competent, and taking into account the present and future incapacity of the respondent, based on a substituted judgment factors enumerated above, that she would consent to the administration of the proposed treatment plan which is offered in good faith by the physician and not for the administrative convenience of the treating facility.

ORDER

IT IS ORDERED THEREFORE that the treatment plan shall be implemented by the treating physician and that the guardian shall have the authority to consent to the treatment by anti-psychotic medication in accordance with the approved plan.

In the event that the purposes of this order are fully accomplished, and the respondent becomes able to give informed consent to medical treatment, a petition to discharge, may be brought at any time.

In the event that a change in the treatment plan is necessary, any party may move to amend said plan at any time.

This order authorizes the guardian to consent to medical treatment, to admit the respondent to a nursing home, and to otherwise authorize treatment in accordance with treatment plan approved herein.

ADDITIONAL FINDINGS ON GUARDIAN'S EXPENSES

1. The respondent is now a resident of a long term care facility and receives MassHealth benefits to pay for her care at said facility.

2. The findings above on Competency and for authority to treat with antipsychotic medication are not repeated but are considered here as applicable.

3. The attorney has presented and certified her fees and costs to obtain the within order and I find said costs to be reasonable and within the amount allowable for payment from the future income of the ward.

FURTHER ORDER ON GUARDIAN'S EXPENSES

IT IS FURTHER ORDERED that $1200.00 is awarded to the Guardian to defray her expenses incurred in establishing MassHealth eligibility for the ward and in obtaining authority to give informed consent to medical treatment for the ward.

_____   _____

Date: Judge of the Probate & Family Court

6-J

Commonwealth of Massachusetts
The Trial Court
Probate and Family Court Department

NOR FOLK **Division**

Docket No. 03 P 1943-G11

In the Matter Of AGATHA T. ADAMS
Of QUINCY
In the County of NORFOLK

NOTICE OF GUARDIANSHIP

To AGATHA T. ADAMS of QUINCY in the County of NORFOLK his heirs apparent or presumptive, a petition has been filed in the above captioned matter alleging that said AGATHA T. ADAMS of QUINCY in the County of NORFOLK is a mentally ill person and praying that REBECCA THATCHER of G. BANNAM in the County of FRANKLIN or some other suitable person be appointed guardian, to serve with personal surety of the person - and property - with the authority to administer antipsychotic medications in accordance with the treatment plan.:

IF YOU DESIRE TO OBJECT THERETO, YOU OR YOUR ATTORNEY MUST FILE A WRITTEN APPEARANCE IN SAID COURT AT DEDHAM ON OR BEFORE TEN O'CLOCK IN THE FORENOON (10:00 AM) ON JULY 28, 2003

WITNESS, HON. FRED CRATER I, ESQUIRE, First Justice of said Court at PEDHAM this day,

Pamela Casey O'Brien

Register of Probate

ORDER OF NOTICE

It is ordered that notice of said proceeding be given by delivering a copy of the foregoing notice in hand to AGATHA T. ADAMS of QUINCY in the County of DEDHAM and by mailing by registered or certified mail a copy of the foregoing citation to all persons interested fourteen days at least before said return date, and if service is made by registered or certified mail, unless it shall appear that all persons interested have received actual notice, by publishing a copy thereof in QUINCY BUGLE, a newspaper published in LYNN: publication to be seven (7) days at least before said return day.

WITNESS, HON. FRED CRATER ESQUIRE, First Justice of said Court, this day,

Pamela Casey O'Brien

Register of Probate

RETURN OF SERVICE

I hereby certify under the penalties of perjury that I have complied with the order of notice by:

[X] serving in hand a copy of the citation as ordered.

[X] mailing - certified - registered - postpaid - a copy of the citation as ordered.

[X] causing the citation to be published in Daily Evening Item, a newspaper published in LYNN.

Publication was on JULY 12 which was at least 7 days/month(s) before said return day.

Date: JULY 25, 2003 Signature: Rebecca Thatcher

6-K

Commonwealth of Massachusetts
The Trial Court

<u>Essex</u> **Division**   Probate and Family Court Department   Docket No. <u>99G1066</u>

TEMPORARY DECREE OF GUARDIANSHIP
GUARDIAN OF PERSON — AND ESTATE

Name of ward <u>AGATHA ADAMS</u>

At a Probate and Family Court held at <u>Salem</u>, on

<u>October 25, 1999</u>,   <u>Judge Phillip Crater</u>, presided.
(date)   (name of justice)

All persons interested having been notified in accordance with the law — Upon an ex-parte motion — and —no objections being made — after hearing — upon representations of counsel, the ward — not — being present:

The Court finds that the situation of the ward which requires emergency attention is <u>the</u>

<u>necessity of establishing authority to give informed consent to</u>
<s>medical care,</s>

and that the petitioners are seeking to avoid the harm of <u>lack of appropriate medical</u>
<u>care in an appropriate setting, i.e., a nursing home</u>

The Court further finds that the ward:

☒   is incapable of taking care of himself/herself by reason of mental illness.

☐   is mentally retarded to the degree that he/she is incapable of making informed decisions with respect to the conduct of his/her — personal —financial affairs and that failure to appoint a guardian would create an unreasonable risk to the ward's health, welfare and property, and that the appointment of a conservator pursuant to G.L.M. c. 201, § 16 would not eliminate the risk.

☐   is unable to make or communicate informed decisions due to physical incapacity or illness.

This temporary guardianship includes:
                                              <u>Long Term Care</u>
☒   authorization to admit or commit the ward to a ~~mental health or mental retardation~~ facility; the action being in the best interest of the ward.

☐   the authority to consent to the following extraordinary medical procedure

_____

_____

_____

CJ-P 114 (10/93)

(BACK OF TEMPORARY GUARDIANSHIP DECREE)

Thus, the Court determines that the welfare of the ward requires the immediate appointment of a temporary guardian and IT IS DECREED that:

Nancy Drew
_____
(name of guardian(1))

10 Downing Street　　Haddonfield　　NJ　　08033
_____
(street address)　　　　　　(city or town)　　　　　(state)　　　(zip code)

~~and~~
_____
(name of guardian(2))

_____
(street address)　　　　　　(city or town)　　　　　(state)　　　(zip code)

be appointed the temporary guardian(s) — of the person — and — the estate — of the ward pursuant to G.L.M. c. 201, § 14. The temporary guardian(s) first giving bond — with — ~~without~~ — sureties for the due performance of said trust.

THE APPOINTMENT OF THIS TEMPORARY GUARDIAN IS LIMITED TO A PERIOD OF NINETY DAYS WHICH EXPIRES ON___January 25, 2000_____.

Date __October 25, 1999___　　　　_____
　　　　　　　　　　　　　　　　　Justice of Probate and Family Court Department

THE APPOINTMENT OF THIS TEMPORARY GUARDIAN IS EXTENDED FOR AN ADDITIONAL NINETY DAY PERIOD AND SHALL EXPIRE ON_____.

Date _____　　_____
　　　　　　　　　　　　　　　　　Justice of Probate and Family Court Department

(The Court may extend for additional ninety (90) day periods the appointment, provided that the affidavit of notice is properly made and an inventory and bond of the temporary fiduciary has been filed in accordance with Probate Court Rule 29B.)

6-L

Commonwealth of Massachusetts
The Trial Court

__Essex__ **Division**   Probate and Family Court Department   Docket No. __99G1066__

PERMANENT DECREE OF GUARDIANSHIP
GUARDIAN OF PERSON — AND ESTATE

Name of ward _____ Agatha Adams _____

At a Probate and Family Court held at ____ Salem _____ , on

__November 30, 1999__ , _____ Judge Phillip Crater _____ presided.
   (date)   (name of justice)

All persons interested having been notified in accordance with the law and — no objections being made — after hearing — upon representations of counsel, the ward — not — being present:

The Court finds that the ward:

☒ is incapable of taking care of himself/herself by reason of mental illness.

☐ is mentally retarded to the degree that he/she is incapable of making informed decisions with respect to the conduct of his/her — personal —financial affairs and that failure to appoint a guardian would create an unreasonable risk to the ward's health, welfare and property, and that the appointment of a conservator pursuant to G.L.M. c. 201, § 16 would not eliminate the risk.

☐ is unable to make or communicate informed decisions due to physical incapacity or illness.

This guardianship includes:

                                        Long Term Care
☒ authorization to admit or commit the ward to a~~mental health or mental retardation~~ facility, the action being in the best interest of the ward.

☐ the authority to consent to the following extraordinary medical procedure

_____

_____

IT IS DECREED that: _____ Nancy Drew _____

__10 Downing Street__   __Haddonfield__   (name of guardian(1)) __NJ__   __08033__
        (street address)   (city or town)   (state)   (zip code)

——xxxxt——————————————————
                              (name of guardian(2))

——————————————————————————————
        (street address)   (city or town)   (state)   (zip code)

be appointed the permanent guardian(s) of the person — and — the estate — of the ward pursuant to G.L.M. c. 201, § 6 — 6A — 6B. The guardian(s) first giving bond — with —xxxxxxxx— sureties for the due performance of said trust.

Date __November 30, 1999__   _____
                                   Justice of Probate and Family Court Department

CJ-P 116 (10/93)

6-M

Commonwealth of Massachusetts
The Trial Court
Probate and Family Court Department

Norfolk Division   Docket No. _03 G 1943_

INVENTORY

To _Rebecca Thatcher_

of _Great Barrington, MA_

Administrator/Administratrix—Executor/Executrix—Trustee—Guardian—
Conservator—Receiver.

YOU are directed to appraise, under the penalties of
perjury, the estate and effects of_____Agatha T. Adams_____
of____Quincy____ which may be in said Commonwealth; and return
to the Probate Court for said County of**_Norfolk_**

_____

Register of Probate Court

Pursuant to the foregoing order to _____ said estate is
appraised as follows:

Amount of Personal Estate,
as per schedule exhibited, _____ $_____

Amount of Real Estate,
as per schedule exhibited, _____ $_____

I—WE—_____
the—trustee—administrator/administratrix—executor/executrix—guard
ian—conservator—receiver—, of the estate of said deceased,
certify under the penalties of perjury that the foregoing is a
true and perfect inventory of all the estate of the within named
that has come to—my—our—possession or knowledge, and sets forth
the actual market values of the various items thereof ascertained
by—me—us—to the best of—my—our—knowledge, information and belief.

_____   _____

_____   _____

_____   _____

Date(s)   Signature(s)

SCHEDULE OF PERSONAL ESTATE IN DETAIL

Dollars   Cts.

Docket No. _____

Inventory

INSTRUCTIONS

Appraise estate as of date of death when filing as administrator, executor, administrator with the will annexed, special administrator, public administrator.

Appraise estate as of date of appointment when filing as conservator, guardian, trustee, receiver.

Inventory—Form CJ-P 41

6-N

COMMONWEALTH OF MASSACHUSETTS

ESSEX, SS
PROBATE AND FAMILY COURT
Docket No. 99- 1066—GI1

In Re: Guardianship of Agatha Adams

MOTION FOR ALLOWANCE OF GUARDIANSHIP EXPENSES

NOW COMES Atticus Finch, attorney for the petitioners,

AND MOVES that this Honorable Court exercise its authority as conferred by G.L. c. 206 § 16 and enter an order consistent with 130 CMR 520.025(E)(3) to award the guardian $1200.00 to defray her expenses incurred in seeking the authority to permit treatment of the ward with anti-psychotic medications, and to otherwise give informed consent to medical treatment, and, further, to order that said award is to be paid from the income of the ward;

AND STATES as reasons for the necessity of such order, that the ward is an indigent person who is hospitalized but needs nursing home placement, and is or will soon be eligible for MassHealth (Medicaid) long term care coverage, and pursuant to the holding in <u>Rudow vs. Commissioner of Division of Medical Assistance</u>, 429 Mass. 218 (March 11, 1999), is entitled to said award for her reasonable costs incurred in obtaining such authority.

FINCH & ABERCROMBY

_____

Date

_____

Atticus Finch

221B Baker Street

Lynn, MA 01902

Tel: 555-9999

BBO #654321

Essex, SS   , 1999

The within motion is hereby allowed/denied.

_____

Judge of the Probate Court

COMMONWEALTH OF MASSACHUSETTS
THE TRIAL COURT
PROBATE AND FAMILY COURT

Essex Division   Docket No. 99-1066—GI1

Statement of Expenses and Services

In the matter of the petition for authorization of the guardian, Nancy Drew, to authorize medical treatment of the ward, and to monitor the administration of anti-psychotic medications to the ward, Agatha Adams.

I, Atticus Finch, hereby certify that I have incurred expenses, the value of which is $160.00, detailed as follows:

Registry of Probate fees	$90.00
Service costs	30.00
Publication in Lynn Item	40.00

and further, that I have performed services the value of which is: $640.00.

Date:	Time:	Nature of services:
10-18-99	1.00	Confer with Nancy Drew, niece of proposed ward
10-19-99	1.20	Prepare guardianship petition and supporting documents, motion for temporary guardian, affidavits
10-21-99	.50	Confer with physician re: medical certificate, correspondence with Probate Court
10-25-99	1.50	Filing petition, hearing on motion for temporary guardian
10-27-99	3.0	Meet with temporary guardian, prepare MassHealth application, review documentation, submit for approval
10-28-99	.50	Attend to service of citation, confer

		with hospital social worker, confer with Eveningtide Nursing Home administrator/social worker
10-29-99	1.50	Confer with Temporary Guardian, who is niece of ward, out of state agent form, MassHealth approval documents
11-30-99	1.20	Hearing re: permanent guardian

Total: 10.40 hours

Billed at $100.00 per hour @ $1040; total costs: $1200.00

Signed under the pains and penalties of perjury.

_____

BBO #

_____   Approved: _____

Date   Justice, Probate & Family Court

6-O

130 CMR: DIVISION OF MEDICAL ASSISTANCE

(c) <u>Guardianship Services Related to the Redetermination Process</u>.

(i) The Division allows a deduction for fees for guardianship services related to the MassHealth redetermination process when the guardian has been appointed by the probate court to assist an incompetent person with securing continued access to medical treatment.

(ii) The Division allows a deduction for reasonable costs related to the MassHealth redetermination process, as approved by the probate court, not to exceed $250. In cases where an administrative hearing is held, the total deduction may not exceed $375 for the costs related to the redetermination process and hearing.

(iii) The deduction is made from the member's monthly patient-paid amount over a 12-month period.

(d) <u>Monthly Guardianship Services</u>.

(i) The Division allows a deduction for monthly fees for a guardian to the extent the guardian's services are essential to consent to medical treatment on behalf of the member.

(ii) The Division allows a deduction, as approved by the probate court, for up to 24 hours per year at a maximum of $50 per hour for guardianship services.

(iii) The Division allows the deduction only if the guardianship services provided include the attendance and participation of the guardian in quarterly care meetings held by the nursing facility where the member lives.

(iv) The Division allows this deduction only if each year the guardian submits to the Division a copy of the affidavit that describes the guardianship services provided to the member.

(v) The deduction is made from the member's monthly patient-paid amount over a 12-month period.

(e) <u>Expenses Incurred by the Guardian in Connection with Monthly Guardianship Services</u>.

(i) The Division allows a deduction up to, but not exceeding, the member's monthly patient-paid amount for filing and court fees incurred by the guardian in connection with monthly guardianship services that are essential to consent to medical treatment for the member.

(ii) If monthly guardianship services are provided, these expenses are included in the affidavit of services required under 130 CMR 520.026(E)(3)(d)(iv).

(iii) The deduction is made from the member's monthly patient-paid amount in the month following receipt of the affidavit of services.

130 CMR: DIVISION OF MEDICAL ASSISTANCE

Trans. by E.L. 63

**MASSHEALTH
FINANCIAL ELIGIBILITY**

Rev. 10/01/99

(5 of 5)

Chapter 520
Page 520.026

(f) Hardship.

(i) If exceptional circumstances exist that make the deductions allowed under 130 CMR 520.026(E) insufficient to cover the expenses required for a guardian to provide essential guardianship services needed to gain access to or consent to medical treatment, the guardian, on behalf of the member, may appeal to the Board of Hearings for an increased deduction.

(ii) A hearing officer may allow for an increased deduction for guardianship expenses only in circumstances where the issues surrounding the member's need to gain access to or consent to medical treatment are extraordinary.

(iii) Extraordinary circumstances may exist when:

1. there is a need for a guardian to consistently spend more than 24 hours per year providing guardianship services to appropriately consent to medical treatment needed by the member; or

2. the circumstances of a MassHealth member cause the guardian appointment or application process to be particularly complex and significantly more costly than the deduction allowed at 130 CMR 520.026(E)(3)(a) or (b).

(g) Guardianship Services and Expenses that are not Deductible. The following fees and costs are not allowed as a deduction under 130 CMR 520.026(E).

(i) Amounts that are also used to reduce a member's assets under 130 CMR 520.004.

(ii) Amounts that are also used to meet a deductible or any other deduction allowed under Division regulations.

(iii) Expenses related to the appointment of a guardian for an applicant when the appointment is made more than six months before submission of a MassHealth application.

(iv) Expenses related to the appointment of a guardian for an applicant or member when the applicant or member does not request a deduction for the appointment within six months of the date of application or date of appointment, whichever is later. However, these expenses may be used as allowed pursuant to 130 CMR 506.010 or 520.032 to meet a deductible.

130 CMR: DIVISION OF MEDICAL ASSISTANCE

Trans. by E.L. 91

MASSHEALTH
FINANCIAL ELIGIBILITY

Rev. 06/21/02

Chapter 520
Page 520.027

(v) Expenses, fees, or costs for expenses that are not essential to obtain medical treatment for the ward including financial management, except when the management is necessary to accurately complete a MassHealth application or redetermination form.

(vi) Expenses, fees, or costs for transportation or travel time.

(vii) Attorney fees, except when payment of the fees is required for the appointment of the guardian.

(viii) Fees for guardianship services provided by a parent, spouse, sibling, or child, even if appointed by the probate court. However, the Division allows a deduction for guardianship expenses in accordance with 130 CMR 520.026(E)(3)(a) and (e).

520.027: Long-Term-Care Deductible

If after applying the deductions in 130 CMR 520.026(A) through (E) the long-term-care-facility resident's monthly income exceeds the public rate at the long-term-care facility, the Division will establish a six-month deductible in accordance with 130 CMR 520.028 through 520.035 and use an income standard of $60.

520.028: Eligibility for a Deductible

The following individuals may establish eligibility by meeting a deductible:

(A) former SSI recipients who are not eligible under the Pickle Amendment;

(B) community-based individuals whose countable-income amount exceeds the 100 percent federal-poverty-level income standards;

(C) long-term-care-facility residents whose income, after general deductions described in 130 CMR 520.026, exceeds the public rate in a long-term-care facility;

(D) disabled adult children whose incomes exceed the standards set forth in 130 CMR 519.004(A); and

(E) persons who are eligible for an increased disregard as described at 130 CMR 520.013(B).

520.029: The Deductible Period

The deductible period is a six-month period that starts on the first day of the month of application or may begin up to three months before the first day of the month of application. The applicant is eligible for this period of retroactivity only if the applicant incurred medical expenses covered by MassHealth and was otherwise eligible.

6-P

10 Downing Street

Great Barrington, MA 02130

Ms. C. DeVille

MassHealth Enrollment Center

21 Spring Street, Suite 4

Taunton, MA 02780

Re: Agatha T. Adams

        Guardianship

        Norfolk Probate Court

        Docket No. 03 P-1943-GI1

Dear Ms. DeVille:

I am writing to inform you that I have been appointed the permanent guardian of my aunt, Agatha T. Adams, by the Norfolk Probate Court.

Enclosed please find copies of:

The decree appointing me as guardian;
The court order stating that the court has allowed costs in the amount of $1,200.00.

As I understand the procedure, you are to revise Agatha's Patient Paid Amount (PPA)—the amount paid to the nursing home—by $100 per month for the next twelve months, so that I may recoup or pay the expenses which I incurred in establishing the guardianship.

Thank you for your courtesy and attention to this request.

Sincerely yours,

Rebecca Thatcher
Tel: (123) 456-7890

6-Q

Commonwealth of Massachusetts
The Trial Court

NORFOLK Division   **Probate and Family Court Department**   Docket No. 03 G 1943

Account

_____FIRST_____ Account of __REBECCA THATCHER__
____GUARDIAN OF THE__ and Estate of _____
__AGATHA T. ADAMS__ as _____
                                        (Specify type of fiduciary and name of estate)

This account is for the period of ____JUNE 1, 2003____ to __MAY 31, 2004__
_____ inclusive.

Principal amounts received per Schedule A $____11,480.00____

Principal payments and charges per Schedule B $____10,210.00____

Principal balance invested per Schedule C $____1,270.00____
   Market value as of _____ per Schedule C $_____
                              (date)

Income received per Schedule D $_____

Payments from income per Schedule E $_____

Income balance per Schedule F $_____

The United States Veterans' Administration is - is not - a party in interest to this account. The ward is - is not - a patient in a State Hospital.

I - We certify under the penalties of perjury that the within account is just and true.

Date____JUNE 10, 2004____   _Rebecca Thatcher_
                                   GUARDIAN OF AGATHA T. ADAMS
                                   _____
                                   Signature of Fiduciary

The undersigned, being _____ interested, having examined the foregoing account, request that the same may be allowed without further notice.

_____
_____
_____
_____

CJ-P 30 (8/88)

For Petitioner:

_____

_____

Tel No. _____

For Respondent:

_____

_____

Tel. No. _____

Publication in the _____

_____

Docket No. _____

Account

Filed _____ 19 _____

Citation Issued _____ 19 _____

Returnable _____ 19 _____

Allowed _____ 19 _____

Recorded Vol. _____ Page _____

Instructions

Refer to Massachusetts General Laws Chapter 206.
(Suggested format for Schedules and use continuation sheets as needed)

SCHEDULE A   shall contain the amount of personal property and with respect to a trustee, guardian or conservator, also the amount of real property, per inventory or balance of principal according to next prior account, and amounts received on account of principal or gains from the sale of any property.

SCHEDULE B   shall contain amounts paid-out and charges on account of principal, losses and distributions of estates.

SCHEDULE C   shall contain the investment of the balance of such account with market values of all assets separately stated. A final account of fiduciary shall contain no balance in this Schedule. Schedule C requires both appraised (book) and market values (P.R. 29A).

SCHEDULE D   trustees only shall report balance of income according to next prior account and amounts received on account of income.

SCHEDULE E   trustees only shall report payments chargeable to income.

SCHEDULE F   trustees only shall report balance of income.

AGATHA T. ADAMS
FIRST ACCOUNT

SCHEDULE A

From Inventory:		1,800.00
Jun 03	SS income	800.00
Jul	"	800.00
Aug	"	800.00
Sep	"	800.00
Oct	"	800.00
Nov	"	800.00
Dec	"	800.00
Jan 04	"	816.00
Feb	"	816.00
Mar	"	816.00
Apr	"	816.00
May	"	816.00
	Total:	11,480.00

SCHEDULE B

Jun 03	Nursing home	640.00
	Guardianship costs	100.00
Jul	Nursing home	640.00
	Guardianship costs	100.00
	Hairdresser (2 months)	40.00
Aug	Nursing home	640.00
	Guardianship costs	100.00
Sep	Nursing home	640.00
	Guardianship costs	100.00
	Hairdresser (2 months)	40.00
Oct	Nursing home	640.00
	Guardianship costs	100.00
	Clothing	60.00
Nov	Nursing home	640.00
	Guardianship costs	100.00
	Hairdresser (2 months)	40.00
Dec	Nursing home	640.00
	Guardianship costs	100.00
	Christmas gifts	80.00
	TV w/ VCR	200.00

Jan 04	Nursing home	756.00
	Guardianship costs	100.00
Feb	Nursing home	756.00
	Guardianship costs	100.00
	Hairdresser (3 month)	60.00
Mar	Nursing home	756.00
	Guardianship costs	100.00
	Clothing	30.00
Apr	Nursing home	756.00
	Guardianship costs	100.00
May	Nursing home	756.00
	Guardianship costs	100.00
	Deposit to funeral trust account	200.00
	Total	10,210.00

SCHEDULE C

Balance	1,270.00

6-R

(A.C. 72)

COMMONWEALTH OF MASSACHUSETTS

To the Honorable the Judges of the Probate Court in and for the County of
  Middlesex:

RESPECTFULLY represents ....
of .... in the County of Middlesex, ...
that by a decree of said Court, dated the .... day of
.... 19 ,   he was adjudged to be
.... and ....
.... of ....
in the County of Middlesex, ... was appointed h................. guardian —
conservator; that said .... accepted the trust
and still continues to have the custody of the person of your petitioner, and the management of h   estate, ...

— that the petitioner ....
has — a — no — wife — husband, whose name is ....
.... of ... .
in the County of .... and as h   only heirs apparent
or presumptive the persons whose names, residences and relationship to h   are as
follows:

NAME	RESIDENCE	RELATIONSHIP

Your petitioner further represents that   he   believes that   he is now capable of
managing h   own estate, that such guardianship—conservatorship is no longer necessary.
Said ward is—not—entitled to any benefit, estate or income paid or payable by or
through the United States Veterans Administration.

Wherefore your petitioner prays that   h   said guardian—conservator may be
discharged.
Dated this .... day of   .... 197 .

The undersigned, relatives, friends and neighbors of the above-named ward, believing
that guardianship — conservatorship of said ward is no longer necessary, hereby concur in
h   petition for h   discharge from said guardianship — conservatorship.

COMMONWEALTH OF MASSACHUSETTS

Middlesex, ss.   PROBATE COURT

At a Probate Court held at Cambridge .... in and for said County

of Middlesex, on the .... day of ....

in the year of our Lord one thousand nine hundred and seventy-..... ....

On the petition of ....

of .... in said County of Middlesex, ...

a person adjudged by said Court ....

and under .... guardianship——conservatorship, representing that such ....

guardianship — conservatorship is no longer necessary, and praying that ....

....

h   guardian — conservator may be discharged from h   said .... guardianship

— conservatorship; ....

It appearing that notice thereof has been given to ....

....

....

and that said petitioner ....

.... is now competent to manage h   estate, and

that such .... guardianship — conservatorship is no longer necessary: ....

It is decreed that said ....

be, and   he is hereby discharged from h   said trust of .... guardian — conserva-

tor of the property of said ward.

.... Judge of Probate Court.

Chapter 7:
Medicaid Rules and Procedures

1.   Why apply for Medicaid?

A central question for any guardian of a nursing home resident will be: How will the nursing home bill be paid? When insurance coverage ceases and savings are depleted, the only sources of payment for nursing home care are the resident's monthly income and a Medicaid subsidy. It is never too early for a guardian to obtain the Medicaid application forms (see Chapter 8, Appendix 8-A) to review the ward's medical conditions and/or needs, and to take an inventory of the ward's assets.

To qualify for Medicaid long-term care coverage, the ward/resident/ applicant must show that:

•   the applicant is financially eligible currently, in terms of income and assets (has income and assets below the allowable amounts, called "standards");

•   the applicant has not transferred (given away without getting full value) assets that result in a disqualification (called a period of ineligibility);

•   the applicant meets the medical criteria established by Medicaid; that is, the ward is sufficiently incapacitated to require a nursing home placement; and

•   the applicant is a citizen or is of eligible alien status. [27]

---

[27] See 130 C.M.R. 518.

2. What are the financial standards or criteria for eligibility for long-term care Medicaid?

    The applicant may have no more than $2,000.00 in COUNTABLE assets and must have monthly income that is less than what Medicaid would pay for the applicant's nursing home care for a one-month period.

3. Are any assets not COUNTABLE?

    Yes, certain assets are not countable:

- a principal place of residence, regardless of whether it is a single-family home or a multi-unit building;

- one motor vehicle;

- some funeral or burial trusts or pre-need contracts into which funds have been pre-paid for funeral arrangements or simply assets (like grave lots or any asset or bank account designated as a funeral asset) worth up to $1,500.00;

- the cash surrender value of life insurance policies if all such policies have a combined face value of less than $1,500.00;

- business and non-business property essential to self support (e.g., rental property) which generates income;

- Loans, grants, the proceeds of the sale of a principal place of residence (for three months after the sale), assets in certain trusts[28], and some lump-sum Social Security or SSI payments, non-countable for six months after receipt. Payments made under a "reverse mortgage" are not income because such payments are loans that must be eventually repaid.

4. What is a countable asset?

    Any asset not mentioned in Question 3 is countable, such as cash, bank deposits, retirement accounts, stocks, bonds, securities, cash surrender value of insurance polices if the face value(s) exceeds

---

[28] Special Needs Trust, Pooled Trusts and ICF/MR trusts—any guardian faced with such issues must consult with an elder law attorney.

$1,500.00, real estate other than the principal place of residence, and assets or income relative to a "Medicaid Qualifying Trust."[29]

A jointly-held bank account is treated as an asset owned entirely by the applicant, and the other joint owner(s) must show that the money does not belong to the applicant in order for such funds to be held non-countable; in other words, the joint owner must show contribution of his or her own funds, in order for Medicaid to treat the bank account as if it is owned proportionately by the applicant and the other joint owner. All other assets are treated as if the applicant owns a proportionate interest. For example, say that Agatha Adams held $20,000.00 in GE stock jointly with her living sister, Tillie. Medicaid would consider that a countable asset worth $10,000.00, that percentage owned by Agatha. If she owned a $20,000 bank account with Tillie, Medicaid says that it is a $20,000 asset unless it can be shown that Tillie contributed her own funds to the account.

5.   Are countable assets ever considered not countable?

Yes, if the applicant has a countable asset that is not accessible (not available to pay for medical bills) and therefore is not available to pay the costs of long-term care, Medicaid will treat the asset as non-countable. For example, suppose Agatha Adams owned a one-half interest in her late mother's home with her sister Tillie who resides in that home. If a joint owner of property states that he or she is unwilling to sell the property, Medicaid will treat the asset as non-countable for as long as the joint owner takes that position. If Ozzie Knellson has a countable asset in just his name, say a bank savings account, and the asset cannot be accessed because he is mentally incapacitated (cannot sign a withdrawal slip or check), Medicaid will treat the asset as inaccessible and give the family six months to obtain a guardianship (or conservatorship, which controls finances only) to access the asset.

---

[29] A Medicaid Qualifying Trust, which should actually be called a Medicaid Disqualifying Trust, refers to a situation where the applicant or his or her spouse created and funded a trust at any time in the past. If the applicant is entitled to any funds from the trust, Medicaid will treat the applicant as if he or she is getting the full entitlement, whether or not the trustee is actually distributing trust funds from the trust to the applicant. See 130 CMR § 520.022(B).

6.   What income is countable?

In long-term care Medicaid, virtually all of the applicant's income is countable: Earned Income includes wages, royalties, and commissions (based on work), and Unearned Income includes Social Security benefits, pensions, annuities, federal Department of Veterans Affairs (VA) benefits, dividends, interest, and net rental income. There are a few examples of income that are not countable income and are specifically exempted, for example, reparations paid to the victims of the Nazis in Germany or income that really amounts to loans (like the payments made by a lender bank pursuant to a reverse mortgage.)[30] Suppose Agatha Adams had her own home, worth $300,000.00, with no mortgage; she has monthly Social Security income of $1000 and is in good health. Her only serious problem is that she cannot meet her monthly living expenses. A reverse mortgage may provide her with the means to remain at home by giving her monthly advances on a mortgage "line of credit" to meet her expenses. Unlike the traditional mortgage, the homeowner does not receive a lump-sum payment that comes with the obligation to make monthly payments. The reverse mortgagor/elder home owner receives agreed upon monthly advances and has no monthly payment obligation. Instead, the balance of the mortgage increases each month, as a result of the payments and the interest due on any balance. The term of the reverse mortgage may be for a period of years, say five or seven, or for the life of the mortgagor. The mortgage must be paid off when the house is sold, or within a stated period of time after the mortgagor ceases to reside in the property. [For free expert advice on reverse mortgages, consult with Homeowners Options for Massachusetts Elders (H. O. M. E.), 37 South Street, Boston, MA 02111, Tel: 617-451-0680.]

7.   What happens if the applicant made a gift (a transfer)?

As part of the application process, Medicaid asks whether the applicant had made any transfer for less than fair market value in the past

---

[30] A reverse mortgage is a potential vehicle for using the equity value in an elder's home to maintain him or her at home. A reverse mortgage may be a way of keeping a frail elder in his or her home where the elder has low income but high equity value in a primary residence.

three years (36 months) and whether the applicant has transferred funds or other assets into or out of any trust in the past five years (60 months). If the answer to either question is yes, Medicaid will ask for the details of such transfers, including documents evidencing the transfer (e.g., deed, bank check) and a copy of any trust(s) documents and all relevant documents, to determine whether the transfer is disqualifying.

If the transfer is disqualifying, Medicaid will impose a period of ineligibility by using the following formula: First, the Medicaid worker determines when the transfer took place and then the value of the asset transferred. The value of the asset(s) transferred is divided by the average cost of one-month, private-pay nursing home care (Medicaid uses $244.00 per day in 2004), to arrive at the number of months for which the applicant will be disqualified. The period of disqualification begins with the month of the transfer.[31] Suppose Agatha Adams gave her nephew Bart a wedding gift of $50,000.00 on November 30, 2003. Since she did not get value, that transfer triggered a penalty—a period of ineligibility for 204 days, or 6.8 month—until July 26, 2004.

8.   Are all transfers disqualifying?

No. The following transfers are not disqualifying: a transfer of a principal residence to or for the benefit of a spouse, a blind, disabled, or minor dependent child, or a "caretaker" child[32] or to a sibling who had an interest and resided in the home for at least one year prior to the nursing home admission of the applicant. Transfers into certain kinds of trusts for the benefit of disabled persons may not be disqualifying

---

[31] As this Handbook was being developed, the Legislature in Massachusetts authorized Medicaid to ask the federal authorities, the Center for Medicare and Medicaid Services (CMS), to permit more stringent rules for transfer of assets penalties. The Medicaid Program has filed such a request, called a waiver, which may change the rules regarding transfer of assets significantly at some time in the future.

[32] A caretaker child is a child who lived with and cared for the applicant in the home that was transferred to the caretaker child for two years prior to the nursing home admission of the applicant, and the care can be shown to have forestalled the nursing home admission.

where the Medicaid rules are followed. An elder law attorney should be consulted regarding trust issues. Countable assets may also be used to purchase annuities for the benefit of the applicant or the applicant's spouse without penalty, but such purchases must be undertaken with expert counsel, to ensure that they comply with Medicaid rules.

9. If a single person like Agatha Adams is permitted to have only $2,000.00 in countable assets, do the same rules apply to Ozzie Knellson, a married man with a "community spouse"?

> Yes and No. Ozzie will not be eligible for Medicaid until he has only $2,000.00 in countable assets held in his name, but there are several protections for Harriet, the community spouse, in terms of how Medicaid treats their income and marital assets in deciding whether or when Ozzie is eligible. A marital asset is any asset held in the names of both spouses, either spouse, or of either spouse with another or other persons. Any jointly held asset with another person is not countable if the joint owner can show contribution, that is, that all or a portion of the jointly owned asset is the property of the other person and not the spouse.

> The first step in evaluating Ozzie's Medicaid application will be for the Medicaid worker to do an "assessment of spousal assets" to determine what were the marital assets as of the date when Ozzie entered the nursing home (sometimes referred to as the "snapshot date"). Then the worker determines which marital assets are going to be Harriet's and which are going to be Ozzie's. Any assets attributed to Ozzie by the assessment must be used for his nursing home costs or for some other permissible purpose. If there are any sizeable assets, an elder law attorney should be consulted.

> If the Knellsons' countable assets add up to less than $18,552.00, Harriet keeps them all, and Ozzie is eligible as of the date of his admission to the nursing home. This is referred to as the minimum community spouse resource allowance.

> If their countable assets add up to twice the minimum ($37,104.00) or greater, the assets are split 50/50, although there is a maximum limit for the community spouse. So, if the couple has $60,000.00 in countable assets, each spouse gets $30,000.00. Ozzie must then spend down his share of the marital assets to the $2,000.000 limit before he becomes eligible for Medicaid coverage. The community

spouse's asset allowance is limited to a maximum of $92,760.00. If they have countable assets of $200,000.00, Harriet gets to keep the maximum of $92,760.00, and Ozzie is allowed $107,240.00, and must spend down to $2,000.00 in order to become eligible.

The Medicaid program will make a determination of spousal assets and send a notice to both spouses. A sample notice appears in Chapter 8, Appendix 8-B.

10.   Can the community spouse ask to keep additional marital assets for his or her support?

Medicaid laws protect a low-income community spouse by the rule relating to the Minimum Monthly Maintenance Needs Allowance (MMMNA).[33] Basically, Medicaid rules provide that the community spouse should not be impoverished by the institutionalization of her spouse. To prevent such a result, she should be permitted to have an income allowance (MMMNA) of up to 150% of the Federal Poverty Level for two persons. In 2004, that figure is $1,515.00. That is the basic allowance. Furthermore, if the community spouse has shelter costs that exceed thirty per cent (30%) of the basic allowance ($455.00), any such excess shelter expenses are added to the basic allowance. Shelter costs include a standard allowance where the community spouse pays for heat and utilities of $425.00 ($258.00 if she does not pay for heat).

Consider Harriet Knellson's case (Chapter 1). She has only $430.00 of monthly income (Social Security benefits). The countable marital assets are $50,000.00. The assessment will put her asset allowance at $25,000.00, which will generate interest income, at 1.8%, or $42.00 monthly[34] Is Harriet's income ($472.00) substantially lower than her MMMNA? She has shelter costs (mortgage, real estate taxes, insurance, utilities) of $620.00 Her MMMNA then is $1,515.00 plus $165.00 ($620.00 minus $455.00) or $1,680.00.

---

[33] 130 C.M.R. 520.026.

[34] Medicaid uses the bank monitor index rate, not actual income earned by the assets, to determine the income attributable to marital assets. See 130 C.M.R. 520.017(c)(3).

There is a shortfall of $1,208.00. Medicaid uses a MMMNA work-sheet to calculate the community spouse's asset allowance, the nursing home spouse's Patient Paid Amount (PPA), and the community spouse's income allowance. See Chapter 8, Appendix 8-C, for a sample worksheet.

Here is how Harriet can bring her income up to her MMMNA:

First, she should request a Medicaid fair hearing and ask for a revised community spouse resource allowance (CSRA). If she can show that she needs additional marital assets to bring her income up to meet her MMMNA, she will be permitted to retain additional assets. She must, however, request a fair hearing. Until September 1, 2003, Medicaid rules permitted the appeal hearing officer to revise the community spouse resource allowance to permit her to retain additional assets to generate additional income to help her meet her MMMNA.[35] Effective with that date, however, Medicaid now uses the "Income First" rule, which means that Mrs. Knellson may not retain additional assets unless her income and her husband's income add up to less than her MMMNA. Because Ozzie's income is $1,280.00, Medicaid now uses his income to defeat her right to retain additional assets, by "deeming" $1,208.00 of his monthly income to her, in order for her income to, at least theoretically, meet her MMMNA.[36] If pending litigation challenging this use of the nursing home spouse's Social Security income is successful, then in the Knellson case, Harriet would be permitted to retain all of the marital assets, because Ozzie's Social Security benefits would not be deemed to her. In a case where all of the marital assets are assigned to Harriet, so that Ozzie is eligible for Medicaid coverage, and her income still does not meet her MMMNA, she has additional rights. Her next step is to request a community spouse monthly income

---

[35] This is called the "Assets First" rule.

[36] There has been litigation filed to challenge the legality of Medicaid's deeming Social Security income of the institutionalized spouse to the community spouse, based on a New York Federal Court of Appeals decision, which held that such a policy violates Social Security law that provides that Social Security benefits may not be involuntarily subject to legal process. Porter v. Waldman, U.S. District Court for Western Massachusetts Docket No. 03-CV-30268.

allowance (CSMIA), that is, the right to retain some of her husband's monthly income to bring her income up to meet her MMMNA. Suppose that Harriet's income, after being permitted to retain all of the marital assets, adds up to only $1,400.00 and her MMMNA is $1,687. Because Ozzie has income of $1,280.00, the hearing officer will permit Harriet to keep $287.00 of Ozzie's monthly income to meet her MMMNA.

So, in the Knellson's case, the community spouse will now not be permitted to retain all $50,000.00 of the marital assets, and Ozzie's share of the assets must be used to meet his nursing home costs. Under the income first rule, she will not be permitted to retain more than her original allowance, because her husband's income will be deemed to her to meet her MMMNA. It is illusory because she will be using assets and income to pay the nursing home bills until her husband's Medicaid eligibility is established. Her only recourse is to purchase an annuity with those assets assigned to her husband and the annuity will provide her with an income stream for the rest of her life. See Question 24 below for a discussion of annuities.

11.   Once a resident becomes Medicaid-eligible, how does Medicaid determine what portion of the resident's monthly income must be paid toward the costs of the resident's care at the nursing home (called the Patient Paid Amount or PPA)?

The resident is notified of Medicaid approval by means of a computer generated notice that explains "the bottom line," that is, the Patient Paid Amount (PPA), the amount of his or her income each month that must be paid over to the nursing home. The notice contains the computation, beginning with the applicant's total countable income, listing any and all deductions or allowances, and arriving at the PPA. A sample of such a notice is found at Chapter 8, Appendix 8-D.

There are several potential allowances or deductions:[37]

•   the personal needs allowance (PNA) of $60.00 for haircuts, slippers, newspapers;[38]

---

[37] The deductions are listed at 130 C.M.R. 520.026.

[38] A veteran or the widow(er) of a veteran has a PNA of $90.00.

- the home maintenance allowance: where a resident has been designated as a short- term stay, that is, for a period of six months or less, Medicaid allows the resident to keep the first $739.00 in monthly income to maintain the home (pay rent, mortgage, etc.), so there will be a home to return to. The amount of the allowance is 100% of the Federal Poverty Level or $739.00 in 2004).

- the community spouse income allowance: where the resident has a community spouse, like Mrs. Knellson, who needs some of the resident's income to meet her MMMNA; the amount of the allowance varies depending on the community spouse's needs).[39]

- a family member's allowance: where there is not only a spouse but other dependent family members of the resident's former household whose income is such that they need some of the resident's monthly income to meet their needs.

- health insurance premiums deduction: where the resident has Medex Silver, there would be a deduction in the amount of the monthly premiums due and payable to Medex each month;

- other medical or remedial expenses: where the resident has medically necessary expenses, which are (a) not covered by health insurance (b) not included in the daily reimbursement rate to the nursing home and (c) not payable if submitted to Medicaid, the resident is entitled to a deduction in order to pay that medical expense. The deduction reduces the payment to the nursing home (the Patient Paid Amount). The allowance results in a reduced PPA but a concomitant increase in the Medicaid subsidy for that month to the nursing home in its subsidy. Medical guardianship costs are one basis for this allowance per the *Rudow* decision.

12. Are there medical criteria an applicant must meet in order to qualify for long-term care Medicaid?

---

[39] There is no allowance for the former spouse of a resident, even where there is a court order for alimony.

To secure Medicaid coverage, the resident must meet the applicable medical criteria, currently so-called "Score 3" criteria; that is, the resident must have at least one skilled nursing care need and must require assistance with at least two activities of daily living.[40] An assessment team from the local ASAP evaluates the resident to determine whether he or she meets the criteria for short-term or long-term placement and documents the findings in a form called an SC-1. A sample is found in Chapter 8, Appendix 8-I.

13. Where can the resident or guardian obtain assistance in applying for long-term care Medicaid?

The Resources section of this Handbook lists elder law projects and contacts for the Massachusetts Chapter of the National Academy of Elder Law Attorneys (NAELA), the Massachusetts Bar Association, and the E.O.E.A.'s SHINE (Serving the Health Information Needs of Elders) program.

14. Who decides whether an applicant is eligible for assistance?

An application is submitted to one of the regional MassHealth Enrollment Centers (See the Resources section). The application is processed by a worker who may request additional information or otherwise ask for supplementation of the application and the documents submitted with it. Any decision of the worker may be appealed but the appeal must be filed at the Board of Hearings within 30 days of the notice of the decision. The hearing is conducted in an informal setting where the hearing officer tries to understand what the decision was and why the appellant is dissatisfied. He or she will issue a written decision in which the Medicaid rules are applied to the case. The hearing officer's decision is appealable to the Superior Court in a complaint for judicial review.[41]

15. What is the spousal waiver program?

---

[40] 130 C.M.R. § 456.409. The Legislature in 2003 authorized Medicaid to apply a "Score 4" criteria prospectively to new nursing home applicants and to retain "Score 3" for current residents. That provision was vetoed by the Governor. The new policy has not yet been implemented because it was anticipated that CMS would not permit a different set of criteria for one population than for another.

[41] M.G.L. c. 30A.

The spousal waiver program is one designed for frail elders who are still in their homes and receiving services from the local Aging Services Access Point (ASAP) and are being cared for by their spouses, but for whom they would be in a nursing home. Generally, if two spouses live in the same household, they must have combined countable assets of less than $3,000.00 in order to be eligible for community (not long-term care) Medicaid. If one spouse is 60 years of age or older, has been evaluated by the ASAP as appropriate to a nursing home placement but can get by at home with help from his or her spouse and ASAP services, then Medicaid will not consider the income or assets of the care giver spouse, but only the assets and income of the frail spouse to determine the latter's Medicaid eligibility. In such a case, Medicaid helps to meet expenses to keep the frail spouse at home because these costs of care are less expensive than if he or she were to be admitted to a nursing home.

If Mrs. Knellson feels that she can manage Ozzie's care at home with Medicaid coverage, she can try to get him back home with spousal waiver eligibility. The ombudsman, the ASAP, and the discharge planner at the facility will help her to explore that possibility.

16. If the nursing home spouse dies before the community spouse, will Medicaid take the home?

When a resident receives the benefit of the Medicaid subsidy for nursing home care, Medicaid keeps a record of all of its expenditures on the resident's behalf. Until recently, if the resident died and left a probate estate (property in just the name of the deceased), then Medicaid would file a claim to recover its costs from the estate of the deceased Medicaid recipient. This is called estate recovery. In 2003, however, the Legislature expanded estate recovery to include "any interest in real and personal property and other assets in which the individual immediately prior to death had any legal title or interest, to the extent of such interest." This includes, "…joint tenancy, tenancy by the entirety, life estate, living trust, right of survivorship, beneficiary designation, or other arrangement." Efforts are currently under way in the Legislature to delay this expansion of estate recovery to July 1, 2004, in order to study its ramifications, which are profound.

It is very important now for Harriet to remove Ozzie's name from the title to any assets, except perhaps the bank account into which his

Social Security benefits are electronically direct deposited. If he dies, Medicaid will seek to recover from his share of the marital home, so she must remove his name from the title. She should consult promptly with an elder law attorney, since the new estate recovery law may also prevent her from refinancing her home.

When the community spouse dies, someone must become the personal representative of the estate and take over the responsibilities of settling the estate. Such circumstances require consultation with an estate attorney to determine promptly what measures should be taken to protect the nursing home spouse or other loved ones of the deceased.

17. What happens when the nursing home resident dies?

Hopefully, the guardian or the family has foreseen the inevitable and has put in place a pre-need funeral contract that reflects the wishes of the individual. A guardian's authority over the ward's affairs ceases at the death of the ward. If there are no pre-paid funeral arrangements in place, there are very limited public funds that may be available to pay for a very modest funeral, not to exceed a payment of $1,100.00, if the costs of the funeral were less than $1,400.00. (See 106 C.M.R. 705.700, 705.710.) There are potential death benefits payable to a surviving spouse by the Social Security Administration or the Department of Veterans Affairs. As discussed above, any property in which the resident had any legal title or interest will be the subject of Medicaid estate recovery.

18. Does the nursing home submit any documentation to Medicaid during the application process?

Yes, the nursing home submits the assessment done by the ASAP team and a statement detailing the resident's admission, the length of stay, and any payments made to the facility since the admission. The nursing home should be informed that a Medicaid application is being filed.

19. What happens if a Medicaid-eligible nursing home resident inherits money?

Any changes in the circumstances of a Medicaid-eligible resident (changes in income, expenses, or assets) must be reported promptly to the Medicaid regional office. The receipt of a substantial inheritance may at least temporarily disqualify a resident from Medicaid coverage and force him or her return to private-pay status. Any guardian who has this experience should consult promptly with an elder law attorney.

20. Once eligible, is a resident's eligibility permanent or is it reviewed later?

A Medicaid recipient or his or her representative must report any financial changes promptly to Medicaid. In addition to a review when such a report occurs, Medicaid conducts its own periodic "re-determinations" wherein the Medicaid office sends forms to the resident or representative, which are to be completed and returned and which describe the resident's financial circumstances. A guardian must respond in a timely manner to such a re-determination request; failure to do so could result in a disqualification and termination of coverage.

21. What happens if a Medicaid-eligible resident moves to another state? Who pays?

A nursing home resident, like all citizens, is free to move to another state if he or she wishes. Generally speaking, a Medicaid-eligible nursing home resident's care is subsidized by the Medicaid Program of the state in which he or she receives the long- term care. The only exception to this rule is where the Medicaid program itself places a resident in another state, in which case the Medicaid program of the original state continues to pay the subsidy.

If Becky moves to Maine after Agatha Adams is established as a Medicaid-eligible nursing home resident in Massachusetts, she would have authority, as Agatha's guardian, to move her to Maine and establish Medicaid eligibility there. The move would involve substantial coordination between the nursing homes and Medicaid Programs involved. Becky should make sure that there are no differences in the Maine Medicaid rules that will cause problems in establishing Agatha's eligibility in that state.

22. What if a Medicaid-eligible nursing home resident is hospitalized and, when ready for discharge, is informed that the nursing home refuses to take him or her back?

A nursing home may not do so. When a nursing home resident is transferred to a hospital for acute care (as distinguished from long-term care), the nursing home must furnish the resident and his or her representative with a form notice of transfer or discharge, which must comply with Medicaid rules.[42] Even a resident who is not Medicaid-eligible must be given such a notice. The notice must inform the resident of the medical reason for the transfer, of the destination of the resident (e.g., the Mercy Hospital), of the facility's "bed-hold" policy, that is, the number of days the bed will be held for the return of a Medicaid-eligible resident. The notice must also inform the resident of the right to appeal the transfer.

When a nursing home refuses to re-admit a resident in such circumstances, the resident or his or her guardian may request a Medicaid appeal hearing (even where the resident is not Medicaid-eligible). Medicaid responds promptly to such appeals and may intervene to require the facility to re-admit the resident pending the appeal. The resident or guardian may also file a complaint with the Abuse Complaint Division of the Department of Public Health (DPH). (See Chapter 2, Question 17.)

23. If a resident owns a primary residence, must it be sold or is a "lien" placed on it?

As long as the resident does not affirmatively declare that the property is no longer his or her residence, Medicaid must treat the home as a non-countable asset. If the resident does declare that the property is no longer his or her home, then it becomes a countable asset and must be put up for sale. Medicaid allows a preliminary term of nine months to accomplish the sale, and that may be extended as long as the recipient or guardian can show that a good faith effort is being made to market the property. The resident or guardian has the option of converting the primary residence to business property by leasing the house to a tenant and making it rent-producing property, which is also a non-countable asset.

A primary residence is also non-countable as long as a spouse, disabled child, or sibling resides in the home.

If the resident owns a primary residence in which no spouse, disabled child, or sibling resides, Medicaid will put a lien on the property.

---

[42] 130 C.M.R. 610.036.

Medicaid files a "notice lien" in the Registry of Deeds in the county where the ownership documents are on record. The purpose of the lien is to inform the world that the owner is a Medicaid recipient and, if and when the property is to be sold, Medicaid will expect to be compensated for its subsidy of the costs of the recipient's care up to the time of the sale. If the resident's name remains on the title to the real estate, then at his or her death, that interest will be subject to Medicaid estate recovery.

24. Can a resident benefit from purchasing an annuity?

Purchasing an annuity involves converting an asset into an income stream. For example, Ozzie Knellson, or his guardian, could take a $50,000 bank account and purchase an annuity from the XYZ Insurance Company, which will pay him or his spouse a monthly sum for the rest of his or her life. In the event that the assessment of assets results in the nursing home spouse's having assets that must be spent on the nursing home costs, Medicaid permits the nursing home spouse to convert those funds to an annuity for the benefit of the community spouse. The guardian should consult with an elder law attorney when considering such action, since there are very strict rules governing annuities. For example, in 2003, the Legislature authorized Medicaid to seek authority to change the annuity rules to provide that any such annuity must name the Medicaid program as the successor beneficiary up to the amount of expenditures paid for the deceased Medicaid enrollee. The rules are so fluid that an expert's guidance is essential in this area.

25. What happens if a nursing home resident has long-term care insurance?

If a resident has been prudent enough to have purchased long-term care (LTC) insurance, the first and most obvious benefit is that some or all of the nursing home costs may be covered by the insurance, which will preserve a resident's individual or marital assets.

Another significant advantage is that if the resident has long-term-care insurance in place upon the date of admission to the nursing

---

[43] See 130 C.M.R. 515.011(B) and the relevant Division of Insurance regulation at 211 C.M.R. 65.09(1)(e)(2).

home and it has the minimum coverage that Medicaid requires,[43] there will be no estate recovery against the estate of the recipient so insured. Suppose that Harriet Knellson were 52 years old, decidedly younger than Ozzie, and her major asset is a primary residence worth $800,00.00, held in her name only. She could ensure that the house will eventually go to her sons or beneficiaries by purchasing long-term care insurance, which would insulate the property from Medicaid estate recovery, even if she were to spend years of Medicaid-subsidized care in a nursing home.

Chapter 8:
The Medicaid Application Process

A guardian or any duly authorized representative of a nursing home resident can obtain the forms for applying for long-term care Medicaid by calling or visiting the nearest MassHealth Enrollment Center. An application form is also available on the DMA website (www.state.ma.us/dma). A list of the Enrollment Centers is found in the Resources section. On request, the guardian will receive a packet containing the application forms and a booklet entitled, "MassHealth and You: A Guide for seniors and persons of any age needing long-term care services." The Guide was prepared by MassHealth, this state's implementation of the federal Medicaid program, and is informational but not advocacy oriented.

Besides the Guide, the packet contains five forms: the Application (red), the Long-Term Care Supplement (blue), the Personal-Care Attendant Supplement (brown), the Appointment of Representative, and the Authorization to Share Information forms. The PCA Supplement form is not relevant to nursing home residents and is used when an individual in the community needs the assistance of a personal care attendant, who comes into the individual's residence and provides personal care (as described in the form). If a guardian is contemplating the ward's discharge from the nursing home and return home, the PCA forms may become relevant as part of the discharge plan.

Copies of the application and other forms appear at the end this chapter, filled out as if the application were being prepared on behalf of Ozzie Knellson by his wife, Harriet. Each question will be discussed to illustrate how a guardian should approach the application process.

As the guardian goes through the application, he or she must recognize that all entries must be documented or supported by written evidence. It is good practice to do a "work copy" and collect all the documents to be submitted before filling out the actual application to be submitted to Medicaid. The guardian should keep copies of the completed application and all documents filed with the application.

An application may be approved retroactively for up to three months. An application filed on May 10, 2004, may be approved with an effective date of February 1, 2004. A guardian must be aware of the ward's outstanding medical bills and may want to submit an incomplete application to preserve a three-month retroactive eligibility date. If assets or even basic information about the value of assets cannot be accessed (e.g., where a Medicaid application is filled but before a guardian is appointed), the applicant or someone on his or her behalf should inform the Medicaid office of the applicant's incapacity. Medicaid rules permit a provisional approval while a guardianship petition is pending.

THE APPLICATION FORM (RED) (Appendix 8-A)

Read the Instructions.

<u>Applicant Information</u>: Enter the information requested.

DOCUMENTATION: copy of birth certificate (or Immigration and Naturalization documents) establishing identity, citizenship, and date/place of birth; if married, copy of marriage certificate; if home is owned, copy of deed; utility bill; if rented, lease or statement of rent being paid; copy of Social Security card; statement from facility regarding the date of admission and any payments made since admission.

<u>Spouse Information</u>: Enter information requested.

DOCUMENTATION: birth certificate, Social Security card; if applicable, statement from facility regarding admission date and payments made since admission.

<u>Previous Medical Bills</u>: Medicaid can approve coverage for up to three months retroactively. An application should state the date of coverage sought. As the forms suggest, the Medicaid worker will tell the guardian what additional information or documentation is needed.

<u>Previous Assistance</u>: If the applicant or spouse was ever on Supplementary Security Income (SSI, which automatically includes Medicaid coverage), enter the details; identify any person assisting the applicant or spouse in paying shelter costs, check appropriate box describing living arrangements.

<u>Personal-Care Attendant Services</u>: Not relevant. Leave blank.

<u>Income from Working</u>: Enter information requested.

DOCUMENTATION: copies of at least two pay stubs for two pay periods; if self-employed, copies of last federal tax return in the forms, it becomes clear that the long-term care application process requires submission of the last two years' income tax returns or, where no returns were filed, a signed form authorizing the IRS to release that information to Medicaid). Rarely does a nursing home resident have work-related income, but the spouse may, and this information is very significant in determining the community spouse's rights to an increased community spouse resource allowance and/or a community spouse income allowance).

Non-Working Income: Enter information requested.

DOCUMENTATION: Medicaid has access to Social Security benefits information, but all other income must be documented; copies of checks or stubs showing gross income and all deductions (e.g., for health or medical insurance coverage). If there is trust income, a copy of the trust instrument must be submitted to show the applicant's interest. A trust created by the applicant or his/her spouse is called Medicaid Qualifying Trust and has special rules (see Chapter 7, endnote 3). The guardian may explain any trust, trust income, or "other" income in a separate letter or affidavit rather than squeeze too much information into the space provided. Rental Income: if there is a tenant living in real estate owned by the applicant or spouse, Medicaid will consider net rental income as available to the applicant or spouse. Submit a copy of the lease, tenant at-will agreement, or a statement from the tenant describing the rent paid, and what utilities are or are not included in the rent payment; bills for all costs related to maintaining the property. Costs related to the rental portion of the property will be used to reduce gross rent to net rent. Bills will show recurring expenses (e.g., real estate taxes). If a repair or maintenance bill is submitted, Medicaid will pro-rate the amount paid over a 12-month period. For example, suppose the applicant just had roof repairs done at a cost of $1,200.00, the amount attributable to the rental-income-producing portion of the property is spread out as a monthly deduction over the next 12 months. Net rental income will appear as part of the computation of the applicant's Patient Paid Amount (PPA), described as "other income."

Health Insurance: Enter information requested.

DOCUMENTATION: Submit copy of Medicare card and all cards showing membership in any health or medical insurance plan (e.g., Medex Gold card). Submit proof of payment of all premiums, including the most recent billing and the check(s) used to pay premiums. If a health or medical insurance plan is paid through deductions from a pension check, indicate such on the form. Any payments made for health or medical insurance will be recognized by

Medicaid, in that the resident will be permitted to retain sufficient monthly income to continue to pay premiums. Medicaid encourages applicants to keep such insurance in place. When Medicaid determines the PPA, a deduction is allowed so that the applicant or guardian can continue to make the premium payments. A guardian may want to cancel such insurance if the community spouse of the nursing home resident can retain the funds as part of his or her community spouse monthly income allowance. In all other cases, the applicant pays either the health insurer or the nursing home, as part of the PPA.

Accident Information: Enter all relevant information. (The purpose of this question is to determine whether the applicant is in a nursing home because of an injury, as from a motor vehicle accident. In such a case, a driver's motor vehicle insurance may cover the costs of any care or treatment required as a result of the injuries; when this happens, Medicaid (and Medicare) may have a lien on any settlement or judgment proceeds recovered against the party responsible for the injuries in any lawsuit brought on behalf of the injured person.)

DOCUMENTATION: Submit the details of the accident, the identity of any attorney representing the applicant, any court cases filed; Medicaid will require that the applicant or guardian sign an agreement to a lien on any settlement or judgment proceeds.

Bank Accounts: Enter all information for bank accounts, open or closed, in the name of the applicant or spouse (whether individually or jointly with another or others) over the last three years. If there is a jointly-owned bank account and in that account are funds that belong to the joint owner, not a spouse, then the applicant must show how the funds are the property of the other joint owner. Upon satisfactory evidence, Medicaid will not count those funds, but they must be removed from the account promptly.

DOCUMENTATION: List all such bank accounts, beginning with currently open ones, identifying the name of the bank, the account number, the type of account (checking, IRA, Certificate of Deposit), the current balance, and balance as of the date the nursing home spouse was admitted to the facility. (This is critical to the calculation of the community spouse's resource allowance.) Identify the name(s) in which the account is held. If there is a joint owner other than a spouse and the joint owner claims that funds in the account are not those of the applicant, submit proof of the claim. For example, say a sibling has his or her Social Security check direct or electronically deposited into the joint account, you must submit a brief history of the account and the percentage owned by the joint owner. The guardian or spouse should take immediate steps to separate the funds of others from those of the applicant.

Once a spouse is found eligible for long-term care Medicaid, all countable assets deemed to the community spouse must be taken out of the name of the nursing home spouse. After 90 days, any asset remaining in the nursing home spouse's name will lead to disqualification if countable assets exceed $2,000.00 in value. All bank account information must be documented with checking account statements, passbooks, or other documents directly from the bank. (This form is for all Medicaid applications, but the long-term care supplement asks about transfers. Identify any transfers, and explain all withdrawals of $1,000.00 or more.) Consider whether to identify any bank account as a funeral asset, which makes the first $1,500 non-countable (list in Prepaid Burial Plans/Trusts section below).

Life Insurance: Enter all information requested.

DOCUMENTATION: Submit the front pages of all life insurance policies to demonstrate the face value. Identify all term policies (they have no cash surrender value). Submit a statement from the insurer of the cash surrender value of each policy. Only the cash surrender value of insurance policies with face values in combination that exceed $1,500 are countable assets. Consider whether to identify an insurance policy as the funeral asset, rather than a bank account. (List in Prepaid Burial Plans/Trusts section. below.)

Trusts: Enter all information if the applicant or spouse created a trust or is the beneficiary of a trust.

DOCUMENTATION: Submit copies of all trust instruments and documents that show transfers into or out of the trust(s) during the previous five years. A trust created by the applicant or spouse is a Medicaid Qualifying Trust. Medicaid treats the applicant who is a beneficiary of such a trust as receiving anything that the trustee has discretion to distribute, whether or not the distributions are being made. A revocable trust created by the applicant or spouse will probably have to be revoked before eligibility can be established. (For example, a primary residence held in a revocable trust will be countable—legal title is in the trust, so not owned by the applicant—until it is transferred back to the name of the applicant or the community spouse.) Any funds received from a trust on a regular basis must be listed in Non-Working Income above.

Prepaid Burial Plans/Trusts: Enter all information requested.

DOCUMENTATION: Submit all documents that relate to funeral contracts and trusts, and include documents that show how such contracts or trusts were funded (e.g., receipts for payments).

Stocks/Bonds/Other: Enter all information requested. Joint owners of stocks and bonds are treated as proportionate owners, and the applicant is deemed to own a fraction of the asset, depending on the number of co-owners: one-half if there are two owners, one-third if there are three owners, etc.

DOCUMENTATION: Copies of bonds, stock certificates, or account statements, etc., which show the value of the asset; if stock certificates, include a stock price quote. If jointly owned, identify the joint owner(s), and include only that portion owned by the applicant as the current value.

Vehicles/Mobile Homes: Enter all information.

DOCUMENTATION: Submit vehicle registration(s) (one motor vehicle is not a countable asset), bill of sale for any mobile home (which should be either a principal place of residence or rental income property, neither of which is a countable asset.)

Annuities: Enter all information requested.

DOCUMENTATION: Submit written evidence of the identities of the owner, the person receiving the income, a copy of the annuity contract, the date purchased and the amount paid. (The purchase of an annuity within the 36-month look-back period for the benefit of the applicant or spouse will not effect eligibility; such a purchase where the beneficiary is another person would trigger a period of ineligibility.)

Real Estate: Enter all information requested.

DOCUMENTATION: Submit copies of deeds (where applicant was the grantee) or estate documents (where applicant inherited real estate) and current tax bills that show the assessed value of the real estate. Explain if the applicant claims that the real estate should not be countable (as when there is a joint owner who refuses to sell the property or where the real estate is business or rental property).

Citizenship: Enter all information if the applicant or spouse is a non-citizen.

DOCUMENTATION: Submit relevant documents, status of INS standing, military discharge, death certificate, court documents related to domestic abuse.

Signature Page: Read and sign. A guardian should submit a copy of the court decree of appointment. An agent under a power of attorney (called an "attorney in fact") should submit a copy of the power of attorney document. Anyone signing the application is doing so under the penalty of perjury and is asserting that all entries are correct and complete to the best of the signer's knowledge.

LONG-TERM CARE SUPPLEMENT FORM (BLUE)

Applicant/Member Information: Enter all information requested.

DOCUMENTATION: If guardianship expenses have been incurred, submit proof of costs or fees paid; where there is community spouse or other dependent family members residing in the applicant's home, submit written documentation of all shelter expenses and income tax returns.

Long-Term Care Insurance: Enter all information requested.

DOCUMENTATION: Submit copy of insurance policy with clear statement of coverage.

Real Estate: Enter all information requested. (This section determines whether or not any real estate is countable, and whether or not a notice lien will be placed on the real estate.)

DOCUMENTATION: Submit all applicable deeds and documents. NOTE: The question, "Do you intend to return to your home?" must be answered very carefully. If the applicant has qualified long-term care insurance, the question must be answered, "no." When the applicant has the requisite long-term care insurance, there will be no estate recovery after his or her death. In all other cases, a "no" answer will render the principal place of residence a countable asset, and Medicaid will require that the property be sold as a condition of approving the application.

Resource Transfers: Enter all information requested. If transfers were made, explain why they should not be the basis for a period of disqualification. If a transfer is indeed disqualifying, find a way to "cure" the transfer (for example, by having the person who received the property give it back to the applicant). If a disqualifying transfer cannot be cured, the applicant or guardian may request a waiver of the period of disqualification in view of the hardship of the applicant.

DOCUMENTATION: If a transfer has been made that will disqualify the applicant for a period of time prospectively, the applicant or guardian must either (a.) "cure" the transfer by getting the assets transferred back to the name of the applicant or spouse, or (b.) claim a hardship, saying, in effect, that the transfer cannot be cured, and it would be inequitable to deny coverage to the applicant under the circumstances of the case. If a transfer has been made that the applicant or guardian claims is permissible, then the necessary documentation must be submitted. For example, suppose that the applicant transferred title of a principal place of residence to a disabled adult child: submit a birth certificate showing the parent-child relationship and a medical certification that the adult child is disabled; a transfer to a caretaker child is documented by submitting a birth certificate and documentation that the caretaker child lived in the residence and provided care to the applicant for at least two years prior to the nursing home admission (statements from the applicant's doctor, ASAP staff, Visiting Nurses' Association, etc.).

Tax Returns: If "yes," submit last two returns. If "no," submit signed Form 4506.

Signature page: Read and sign.

Appointment of Representative Form

Because of privacy issues, Medicaid will deal only with the applicant or his or her duly authorized representative. The form must be filed out and signed and submitted with the application.

Authorization to Share Information Form

As a result of the health and medical privacy provisions of federal law (The Health Insurance Portability and Accountability Act or HIPAA), Medicaid requires that the DMA workers be given authority by the applicant or representative to discuss and disclose information regarding the applicant's health and medical issues, when appropriate. This form must be filled out and signed and submitted with the application.

Filing the Application

Once the application is completed and the documentation, as best as can be done, has been collected, the application with documentation must be filed at a regional MassHealth Enrollment Center. It is recommended that the application be filed in person, although it can be sent by mail. If the application is filed in person, a worker will review the documents with the guardian and may request additional documents. The worker will give the guardian a list of what additional documents are required. If the application is mailed, the Medicaid worker will mail such a request (see sample at Appendix 8-E). Sometimes a request for more information is really a denial (see sample at Appendix 8-F). A guardian must be careful to appeal any adverse decisions, where documentation is lacking, if the applicant needs retroactive coverage. The right to make another application later is very different from the right to appeal. **Only an appeal, filed within 30 days of the denial of coverage, will preserve the applicant's right to the retroactive coverage requested in the application.**

When the worker is satisfied that all the necessary documentation is submitted, a decision is made, either approval (sample at Appendix 8-D) or a denial (sample at Appendix 8-F).

An approval will reflect the applicant's income, deductions, Patient Paid Amount, and the start date of eligibility.

When the applicant has a community spouse, additional documents are generated. An assessment of marital assets (sample at Appendix 8-B) and a spousal notice supplement and monthly maintenance needs allowance worksheet (sample at Appendix 8-C) must be completed. Those forms tell the community spouse about his or her rights with respect to marital resources and the right to appeal any decision in order to increase his or her resource allowance and to request a community spouse monthly income allowance. In many cases, a community spouse will appeal a decision, if he or she is entitled to an increased resource or income allowance.

Appealing a Medicaid Decision

Every Medicaid decision should be in writing, should clearly inform the applicant or guardian of the meaning of the decision, and should explain that any person aggrieved by the decision has the right to appeal. In most cases, the appeal form is on the reverse side of the decision itself (see sample at Appendix 8-G).

An appeal must be filed within 30 days of the receipt of the decision. The 30 days begin with the date of the decision plus five days to allow for mailing. Appeals may be mailed to the Board of Hearings (BOH), Two Boylston Street, Boston, MA 02116 or may be faxed to the BOH at 617- 210-5820.

The guardian must be prepared to show the appeal hearing officer why the decision was wrong. Assistance with such an appeal is usually available from the local federally funded elder law project (see list in the Resources section). Experienced advocates often prepare a memorandum of fact and law for submission to the appeal hearing officer. A sample of such a memorandum, where Mrs. Knellson is appealing the community spouse resource allowance, is at Appendix 8-H.

The appeal hearing officer will give at least ten (10) days advance notice of the hearing date, time, and place. The hearing will be conducted "informally" in that strict rules of evidence do not apply. The hearing officer reviews the procedure and explains why the parties are present. When everyone is ready to begin, the hearing officer turns on a tape recorder and begins the hearing. The proceedings are recorded because the appellant has the right of further appeal (to the Superior Court in a proceeding called a "complaint for judicial review") and the tape is the official record of the proceedings. The hearing officer requests that all present identify themselves for the record (so that later, if necessary, a transcriber can follow and prepare a transcript of what was said at the hearing) and then reviews what documents are in the record. The record usually consists of copies of the application, the denial, and the appeal request. The hearing officer typically marks these documents respectively as Exhibit 1, Exhibit 2, and Exhibit 3. The Medicaid worker is then called upon to explain the decision. The hearing officer will ask questions and may put additional documents into the record. Next, the hearing officer permits the applicant or the applicant's representative to ask questions of the worker. Then, the hearing officer questions the appellant or the representative and will permit the worker to ask any questions of the appellant, the representative, or any witnesses. Once the hearing officer is satisfied that everything that should be on the record has been included, either by testimony or by the Exhibits, the hearing is closed.

A written decision is issued in due course, and, if adverse, the appellant may request a Commissioner's review (130 C.M.R. 610.091) within 14 days or file a complaint for judicial review within 30 days.

A guardian is not begging for the ward but performing a legal duty to assert the ward's legal rights and entitlement to Medicaid benefits. A guardian who is apprehensive about the appeal process should confer with counsel. Most free elder legal services programs would treat such a case as a priority.

Appendices to Chapter 8

8-A

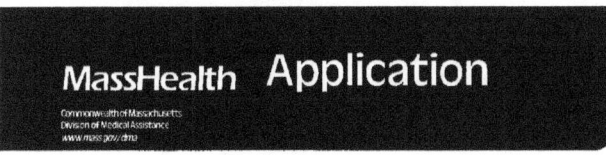

Instructions

Please read these instructions before you fill out the MassHealth Application.

Dear Applicant:

You must fill out the enclosed MassHealth Application (red form) to apply for MassHealth if you live in Massachusetts and:

- are aged 65 and older and living at home;
- are any age and need long-term-care services in a medical institution; or
- are eligible under certain programs to get long-term-care services to live at home.

You will also need to fill out the Long-Term-Care Supplement (blue form) if you are:

- in an institution, like a nursing home, chronic hospital, or other medical institution; or
- in an acute hospital waiting for placement in a long-term-care facility.

If you are aged 60 and older and need long-term-care services to live at home, you may also need to fill out the Long-Term-Care Supplement. We will let you know.

After your application is filled out and reviewed, **you will be given the most complete coverage that you qualify for.**

There is a different application for you if you are:

- any age and both disabled and working 40 or more hours a month;
- under age 65 and not in a medical institution, and you do not need long-term-care services; or
- aged 65 or older and a parent or caretaker relative of children under age 19.

To get this other application, called a Medical Benefit Request (MBR), call the MassHealth Customer Service Center at **1-800-841-2900** (TTY: 1-800-497-4648 for people with partial or total hearing loss).

This application package contains:

- a MassHealth Application (red form)
- a Long-Term-Care Supplement (blue form) (including IRS Form 4506)
- a Personal-Care Attendant Supplement (gold form)
- a Primary Language Identification Form
- information about voter registration (You do not need to register to vote to get MassHealth.)
- the "MassHealth and You" guide, which explains who is eligible for MassHealth, what the income and asset rules are, what medical services you can get under MassHealth, and what your rights and responsibilities are
- a MassHealth Eligibility Representative Designation Form (If you want someone to act on your behalf, you can use this form to tell us who this person is.)

MHA (Rev. 04/03)   *-over*

When you fill out the MassHealth Application, remember to:

- **Read carefully the "MassHealth and You" guide before you fill out the application. Keep the guide. It may answer questions you have later.**

- Answer all questions and fill out all sections on the application and on any supplements. If you need more space, use a separate sheet of paper, and attach it to the application.

- **Send proof of all current income before deductions,** like copies of pension check stubs. (You do not have to send proof of social security income.)

- **Send proof of all assets,** like bank accounts and life insurance policies.

- If you or your spouse who is applying is not a U.S. citizen, send a copy of both sides of all immigration cards (or other documents that show immigration status).

- Send a copy of both sides of **all** health-insurance cards for those who are applying, and copies of current premium bills. (You do not have to send copies of your Medicare cards.)

- **Sign and date all the forms after you finish filling them out.** If you are married, your spouse must also sign.

- Submit a filled-out MassHealth Eligibility Representative Designation Form, if you are filling out this application as an eligibility representative or if you want someone to act on your behalf.

- After you have filled out the MassHealth Application (MHA) and any needed supplements, **send** the filled-out MHA, any supplements, and any needed papers **to the one MassHealth Enrollment Center (MEC) listed below that is closest to where you live.**

Revere MEC	**Taunton MEC**
300 Ocean Avenue	**21 Spring Street**
Suite 4000	**Suite 4**
Revere, MA 02151	**Taunton, MA 02780**
Springfield MEC	**Tewksbury MEC**
333 Bridge Street	**367 East Street**
Springfield, MA 01103	**Tewksbury, MA 01876**

If you need more information about how to apply, or if you need another copy of the Long-Term-Care Supplement or Personal-Care Attendant Supplement for your spouse who is also applying, call the MassHealth Customer Service Center at **1-800-841-2900** (TTY: 1-800-497-4648 for people with partial or total hearing loss).

If you want us to share information about your MassHealth eligibility (including copies of notices we send you) with someone other than your Eligibility Representative, if you have one, please call MassHealth. MassHealth can give you a MassHealth Permission to Share Information form.

If you have any questions about any form or the information you need to send, please call a MassHealth Enrollment Center at **1-888-665-9993** (TTY: 1-888-665-9997 for people with partial or total hearing loss).

Nonworking Income

▶ Do you or your spouse have any other income, including rental income? .... ☒ yes ☐ no
  If **no**, go to page 4 *(Health Insurance)*.
  If **yes**, fill out this section, and the rest of this page *(Rental Income)*.

✉ **Send proof** of income before deductions (for example: check stub or award letter). (You do not have to send us proof of social security income.)

	You Monthly amount before deductions	Your spouse Monthly amount before deductions
Social Security/Railroad Retirement	$ 860	$ 430
Veterans' benefits (state or federal)	$	$
Retirement/Pension G.E. PENSION	$ 420	$
Annuity	$	$
Dividend/Interest	$	$
Trust income	$	$
Other (identify:)	$	$

▶ If you have **rental income** from any real estate, including your home, fill out this section.

✉ **Send proof** of current rental income, like a written statement from each tenant or a copy of the lease, or a current federal tax return.

✉ **Send proof** of all of the following expenses, if applicable, for the last 12 months:
  • mortgage   • taxes   • utilities (gas/electric)   • heat
  • water/sewer   • insurance   • condo or co-op fee   • repairs and maintenance

▶ What type of real estate do you own?
  ☐ one-family   ☐ two-family   ☐ three-family   ☐ other (describe: _____)

▶ How much monthly rental income do you get from each rental unit from the real estate indicated above? (List each rental unit and address separately.)

Address: _____ Unit #: _____ Amount: $ _____

Address: _____ Unit #: _____ Amount: $ _____

▶ Do you pay for heat and/or utilities for your tenant? .... ☐ yes ☐ no

Health Insurance

▶ **Medicare:** Do you or your spouse have Medicare? .... ☒ yes ☐ no

▶ **Medicare supplemental insurance:** Do you or your spouse have supplemental health insurance (like Medex or AARP)? .... ☒ yes ☐ no

▶ **Other health insurance:** Do you, your spouse, or former spouse have other health insurance? .... ☐ yes ☐ no
   If you answered no to all of these questions, go to the next section (Accident Information).
   If you answered yes to any of these questions, fill out this section.

✉ **Send a copy** of both sides of all health-insurance cards, and copies of your current premium bills. (You do not have to send us copies of your Medicare cards.)

✉ **Send a copy** of the policy if you have long-term-care insurance.

	You	Your spouse
Insurance company name *MASS BC/BS*	**394.53**	**394.53**
Policy number *MEDEX 3 - 21828*		
Policy start date *?*	/ /	/ /
Insurance company name		
Group number		
Policy start date	/ / .	/ /
Policyholder name		
Policyholder date of birth	/ /	/ /
Policyholder social security number		
Policy type	☐ individual ☐ couple *(2 adults)* ☐ family	☐ individual ☐ couple *(2 adults)* ☐ family

Accident Information

▶ Are you or your spouse applying because of an accident or injury that someone else might be responsible for? .... ☐ yes ☒ no

▶ Do you or your spouse have an injury, illness, or disability that was caused by someone else, or that could be covered by someone else's insurance or your or your spouse's own insurance other than health insurance (like homeowner's or auto insurance)? .... ☐ yes ☒ no

▶ Has a lawsuit, a worker's compensation claim, or an insurance claim been filed for you or your spouse as a result of an accident, illness, or injury? .... ☐ yes ☒ no

4.

Instructions for telling us about your assets

You must fill out all blocks for each asset you or your spouse own. If you are applying for long-term care, you must *also* give us information about all assets you or your spouse owned in the last 36 months. If you have a spouse at home, also fill out the shaded blocks*. If you need more space, please use a separate sheet of paper, and attach it to this application.

Bank Accounts

▶ Do you or your spouse have any bank accounts or certificates of deposit, including checking, savings, personal needs account (PNA), credit union, NOW, and money-market accounts? .... ☒ yes ☐ no

▶ Do you or your spouse have any retirement accounts, including individual retirement accounts (IRAs), Keogh accounts, or pension funds? .... ☐ yes ☒ no

▶ Have you or your spouse or a joint owner closed any accounts in the last 36 months, including any accounts you had owned jointly with anyone else? .... ☐ yes ☒ no

*If you answered **no** to **all** of these questions, go to the next section (Life Insurance).*
*If you answered **yes** to **any** of these questions, fill out this section.*

☒ **Send a copy** of your passbooks updated within the last 45 days and/or a copy of your current account statements.

Name on account	Name of bank/institution	Account number	Account type
OSWALD AND HARRIET KNELLSON	HUGELY BANK	987654-0	CHECKING
Current balance $ 1201.00	☒ account open ☐ account closed	Date account closed / /	Balance on admission date* $ 1651.00
OSWALD AND HARRIET KNELLSON	BOSTON SAVINGS BANK	1246810	CD
Current balance $ 20,210.00	☐ account open ☐ account closed	Date account closed / /	Balance on admission date* $ 20,201.00
OSWALD AND HARRIET KNELLSON	TOWN SAVINGS BANK	10987-01	SAVINGS
Current balance $ 18,020.00	☐ account open ☐ account closed	Date account closed / /	Balance on admission date* $ 18,016.50
Name on account	Name of bank/institution	Account number	Account type
Current balance $	☐ account open ☐ account closed	Date account closed / /	Balance on admission date* $
Name on account	Name of bank/institution	Account number	Account type
Current balance $	☐ account open ☐ account closed	Date account closed / /	Balance on admission date* $
Name on account	Name of bank/institution	Account number	Account type
Current balance $	☐ account open ☐ account closed	Date account closed / /	Balance on admission date* $

*Enter the account balance you had on the date of admission to medical institution.

5.

Life Insurance

▶ Do you or your spouse have any life insurance? .... ☒ yes ☐ no
  If **no**, go to the next section *(Trusts)*.
  If **yes**, fill out this section.

✉ **Send a copy** of the first page of all life insurance policies. If total face value of all policies exceeds $1,500 per person, also send a letter from the insurance company showing the current cash-surrender value (for all policies except term policies).

Name of insured person	Insurance company	Policy number	Face value
OSWALD KNELLSON	METLIFE	998999	$5000.00
HARRIET KNELLSON	METLIFE	212122	$2000.00
			$

Trusts

▶ Are you or your spouse the grantor, trustee, or beneficiary of any trust(s)? .... ☐ yes ☒ no

▶ Have you, your spouse, or someone else on your behalf contributed income or assets owned by you or
  your spouse to a trust? .... ☐ yes ☒ no

▶ Are you or your spouse a beneficiary of a trust established by someone else, including a court, administrative
  body, or any other person? .... ☐ yes ☒ no
  If you answered **no** to **all** of these questions, go to the next section *(Prepaid Burial Plans/Trusts)*.
  If you answered **yes** to **any** of these questions, fill out this section.

✉ **Send a copy** of the trust document(s) showing financial activity and the schedule of beneficiaries.

Name of trust	Irrevocable?	Trustee(s)	Grantor(s)	Beneficiaries	Current trust principal	Trust principal on admission date*
	☐ yes ☐ no				$	
	☐ yes ☐ no				$	
	☐ yes ☐ no				$	
	☐ yes ☐ no				$	

Prepaid Burial Plans/Trusts

▶ Do you or your spouse have any prepaid burial contracts or trusts, life insurance set up for funeral and burial expenses, or
  bank accounts set aside for funeral and burial expenses? .... ☐ yes ☒ no
  If **no**, go to the next section *(Stocks/Bonds/Other)*.
  If **yes**, fill out this section.

✉ **Send a copy** of the trust contract, trust instrument, insurance policy, or burial-only account.

	You		Your spouse	
Burial contract	☐ yes (amount: $	) ☐ no	☐ yes (amount: $	) ☐ no
Burial trust	☐ yes (amount: $	) ☐ no	☐ yes (amount: $	) ☐ no
Life insurance for burial	☐ yes (total face value: $	) ☐ no	☐ yes (total face value: $	) ☐ no
Burial-only account	☐ yes (amount: $	) ☐ no	☐ yes (amount: $	) ☐ no

*Enter the trust principal you had on the date of admission to medical institution.

6.

Stocks/Bonds/Other

▶ Have you, your spouse, or someone acting on your behalf given a deposit to any health-care or residential facility, like an assisted-living facility?.. ☐ yes ☒ no

If yes, give us the name and address of the facility, the amount of the deposit, and the date it was given to the facility.

✉ **Send a copy** of the documents.

Name of facility	Address of facility	Amount	Date
		$	/ /

▶ Do you or your spouse own any stocks, bonds, savings bonds, mutual funds, securities, assets held in safe-deposit boxes, or cash not in the bank?.. ☐ yes ☒ no

If no, go to the next section *(Vehicles/Mobile Homes)*.

If yes, fill out this section.

✉ **Send a copy** of the documents.

	You			Your spouse		
	Company	Current value	Value on admission date*	Company	Current value	Value on admission date*
Stocks		$			$	
Bonds		$			$	
Savings bonds		$			$	
Mutual funds		$			$	
Securities		$			$	
Other		$			$	

Vehicles/Mobile Homes

▶ Do you or your spouse own any vehicles, including cars, vans, trucks, recreational vehicles, mobile homes, and boats? ☒ yes ☐ no

If no, go to the next section *(Annuities)*.

If yes, fill out this section.

✉ **Send a copy** of the registration for each vehicle, and proof of the outstanding loan balance. For mobile homes, **send a copy** of the bill of sale. If you have a spouse at home, **send proof** of the fair-market value of each vehicle as of the date of admission to the medical institution.

	You	Your spouse
Type of vehicle		MERCURY SABLE
Year/make/model		1998
Fair-market value	$	$ 1000.00
Amount owed	$	$ Ø

*Enter the account balance you had on the date of admission to medical institution.

7.

Annuities

▶ Do you or your spouse own an annuity? .... ☐ yes ☒ no
If no, go to the next section *(Real Estate).*
If yes, fill out this section.

✉ **Send a copy** of the contract.

	You	Your spouse
Name of owner		
Name of person getting income		
Date purchased	/ /	/ /
Amount (purchase price)	$	$

Real Estate

▶ Do you or your spouse own or have a legal interest in any real estate other than your primary residence, including a life estate? .... ☐ yes ☒ no
If no, go to the next section *(Citizenship).*
If yes, fill out this section.

✉ **Send a copy** of the deed(s) and current tax bill(s).

Address	Type of property

Citizenship

▶ *If you and your spouse are U.S. citizens*, you do not have to fill out the rest of this page. Go to page 10.
▶ *If you or your spouse are not U.S. citizens*, and you are applying, you must fill out the rest of this page.

1. Are you or your spouse a veteran of the United States Armed Forces with an honorable discharge
   or did you or your spouse serve under U.S. command during World War II or in Vietnam?............................ ☐ yes ☐ no
   If yes, you may stop here and go to page 10.
   If no, go to the next question.

2. Are you or your spouse the widow or widower of a veteran described above? .... ☐ yes ☐ no
   If yes, you may stop here and go to page 10.
   If no, go to the next question.

3. Are you a victim of domestic abuse and **no longer living with the abuser**?................................. ☐ yes ☐ no
   If yes, you may stop here and go to page 10.
   If no, you must fill out the rest of this page *(Immigration Status)*.

▶ List *all* statuses that have applied to you or your spouse since entering the U.S.

✉ **Send copies** of both sides of all immigration cards (or other documents that show immigration status).

Note: If you and your spouse are applying only for MassHealth Limited, you do not have to give us a social security number. We will not match your names with any other agency including the Department of Homeland Security (DHS). You do not have to list your names on this page or send proof of your immigration status. MassHealth Limited pays for emergency services only.

Use these codes to describe your status in the chart below.

4. Amerasian admitted pursuant to Section 584 of Public Law 100-202	5. Granted asylum 6. Conditional entrant 7. Cuban/Haitian entrant	8. Deportation withheld 9. Legal permanent resident 10. Native American with at least 50% American Indian blood born in Canada	11. Granted parole 12. Refugee 13. Person with a temporary visa/other 14. Person residing under color of law (PRUCOL)

Name	Status codes (List all that apply.)				Date status awarded				U.S. entry date
	a	b	c	d	a	b	c	d	
									/ /
									/ /

You, your spouse, and/or your eligibility representatives must read this page carefully, then sign and date it at the bottom.

I give permission for my current and former employers and health insurers to release to the Division any and all information they have about my health-insurance coverage and health-insurance coverage for my spouse. This includes, but is not limited to, information about policies, premiums, coinsurance, deductibles, and covered benefits that are, may be, or should have been available to me or my spouse.

I give permission to the Division to get any records or data to prove any information given on this application and any supplements, or other information I give to the Division once I am a member. If I or my spouse is found eligible for MassHealth, I give permission to the Division to get any records about medical services provided through MassHealth.

I understand that in some cases, the Division may place a lien against any real estate that I have a legal interest in. If the Division puts a lien against my property and I sell it, I may need to use money I get from the sale of that property to repay the Division for medical services that I get.

I understand that after I die, the Division may be able to get money from my probate estate. I understand that the "MassHealth and You" guide has important additional information about the Division's recovery rules and exceptions to these rules.

I understand that if I or my spouse is in an accident, or we are injured in some other way, and get money from a third party because of that accident or injury, we will need to use that money to repay the Division for certain medical services provided, as explained in the "MassHealth and You" guide. I also understand that I must tell the Division in writing, within 10 days, if I or my spouse files any insurance claim or lawsuit because of an accident or injury to me or my spouse.

I understand that if I or my spouse is eligible for MassHealth, I must tell the Division of any changes in my or my spouse's income or employment, assets, health-insurance coverage, and health-insurance premiums, or of changes in any other information I gave on this application and any supplements within 10 days of learning of the change.

I also understand that by signing below, I give permission to the Division to go after and collect third-party payments for medical care and medical support from my spouse who is living at home and refuses to cooperate or whose whereabouts is unknown.

I certify that I have read or had read to me the information on this application and the information in the "MassHealth and You" guide, and that I understand my rights and responsibilities. I further certify under penalty of perjury that the information on this application is correct and complete to the best of my knowledge.

If you are acting on behalf of someone in filling out this application, the enclosed MassHealth Eligibility Representative Designation Form must also be filled out and sent back with this application. Your signature on this application as an eligibility representative certifies that the information on this application is correct and complete to the best of your knowledge.

If you think the Division's decision about whether you are eligible is wrong, you have the right to appeal. If you are denied benefits, you will get information on how to appeal.

X *Harriet M. Knellson*   JUNE 8, 2003
Signature of applicant or eligibility representative   Date

X
Signature of applicant's spouse or spouse's eligibility representative   Date

10.

MassHealth Long-Term-Care Supplement

Commonwealth of Massachusetts
Division of Medical Assistance
www.mass.gov/dma

Please read the "MassHealth and You" guide carefully before you fill out this supplement. If you are applying for MassHealth and need long-term-care services, fill out this supplement (blue form) and the MassHealth Application (red form). If you are already a MassHealth member and applying for long-term-care services, fill out this supplement (blue form) and a MassHealth Eligibility Review form (green form).

Please print clearly. Answer all questions and fill out all sections. If you need more space to finish any section, please use a separate sheet of paper, and attach it to this supplement.

Applicant/Member Information

Last name KNELLSON	First name OSWALD	MI J.	Social security number 030-30-9999

▶ Do you have to pay guardianship expenses for a court-appointed guardian?.. ☒ yes ☐ no

Your spouse living at home may be able to keep some of your income. Fill out the following information about your spouse's current living expenses.
If you do not have a spouse, go to the next section (Long-Term-Care Insurance).

▣ **Send proof** of your spouse's current living expenses.

▶ 1. How much does your spouse pay each month for:

Rent?	Mortgage (principal and interest)?	Homeowner's/ tenant's insurance?	Real estate taxes?	Required maintenance charge for a condo or co-op?	Room and board for assisted living?
$ —	$ 520.00	$ 110.00	$ 130.00	$ —	$ —

▶ 2. Does your spouse pay for heat? .... ☒ yes ☐ no

▶ 3. Does your spouse pay for utilities? .... ☒ yes ☐ no

▶ 4. Is a child, parent, brother, and/or sister living with your spouse? .... ☐ yes ☒ no
If no, go to the next section (Long-Term-Care Insurance).
If yes, fill out this section.

▣ **Send proof** of their monthly income before deductions.

A deduction may be allowed for their maintenance needs. These persons must be related to you or your spouse, and one of you must claim them as dependents on your federal income tax return.

Name	Social security number	Relationship	Date of birth	Monthly amount before deductions
HARRIET KNELLSON	301-30-1234	SPOUSE	1 / 15 / 24	$ 430
			/ /	$

Long-Term-Care Insurance

▶ Do you or your spouse have long-term-care insurance? .... ☐ yes ☒ no
If no, go to the next section (Real Estate).
If yes, fill out this section.

▣ **Send a copy** of the policy.

Policy number	Policyholder name	Effective date	Premium amount
		/ /	$
		/ /	$

LTC-SUPP (Rev. 04/03)

Real Estate

The answers to the following questions will be used to decide if: (1) your real estate will be counted as an asset; or (2) a lien will be placed against your real estate. Your home is a noncountable asset if you intend to return to it. Your home may be subject to a lien. However, if you own long-term-care insurance that meets certain requirements when you enter a long-term-care facility, your home is noncountable regardless of your intent to return.

▶ 1. Do you or your spouse own or have a legal interest in your home, including a life estate? .... ☒ yes ☐ no
If yes, fill out the following information and answer questions 2 through 4.
If no, answer question 4 only.

Name and address of person(s) on ownership papers	Description and address of property location	Fair-market value
OSWALD AND HARRIET KNELLSON	PRIMARY RESIDENCE – SINGLE FAMILY HOME AT 123 CLOVER CIRCLE, DORCH.	$ $ 180,000.

2. Do you have a	*If you answered yes,* fill out this column and the next. ☛	Is this person living in your home?
Spouse?	Name: HARRIET	☒ yes ☐ no
Permanently and totally disabled or blind child? ☐ yes ☐ no	Name:	☐ yes ☒ no
Child under 21 years of age? ☐ yes ☐ no	Name: Date of birth: / /	☐ yes ☒ no
Brother or sister with a legal interest in the home who was living in the home for at least one year immediately before your admission to the medical institution? ☐ yes ☐ no	Name:	☐ yes ☒ no
Son or daughter who has lived in the home for at least the last two years before your admission to the medical institution and has provided care to you that allowed you to live in the home? ☐ yes ☐ no	Name:	☐ yes ☒ no
Dependent relative? ☐ yes ☐ no	Name: Describe the relationship and the nature of the dependency:	☐ yes ☒ no

Spouse? ☒ yes ☐ no

▶ 3. Do you intend to return to your home? .... ☒ yes ☐ no

▶ 4. Do you or your spouse own or have a legal interest in other real estate not listed in #1 above? .... ☐ yes ☒ no
If yes, please describe the property and list its address below.

_____

_____

_____

_____

Resource Transfers (resources include both income and assets)

▶ 1. In the last 36 months:

    a. Did you, your spouse, or someone on your behalf transfer income or the right to income?.................................... ☐ yes ☒ no

    b. Did you, your spouse, or someone on your behalf transfer, change ownership in, give away, or sell any assets, including your home or other real estate? .... ☐ yes ☒ no

    c. Did you, your spouse, or someone on your behalf change the deed or the ownership of any real estate, including creating a life estate? .... ☐ yes ☒ no

    d. Did you, your spouse, or someone on your behalf add another name to the deed of any property you own?......... ☐ yes ☒ no

    e. Did you, your spouse, or someone on your behalf give anyone a mortgage or promissory note on property you own? .... ☐ yes ☒ no

▶ 2. In the last 60 months, has any property available or belonging to you or your spouse been transferred into or out of a trust of which you or your spouse are or had been a beneficiary, trustee, or grantor? .... ☐ yes ☒ no

*If you answered **yes** to any of the questions above, you must fill out the following.*

Description of asset/income	Dates of transfer	Transferred to whom	Relationship to you or your spouse	Amount of transfer
	/ /			$
	/ /			$
	/ /			$

▶ 3. Have you, your spouse, or someone acting on your behalf given a deposit to any health-care or residential facility, like an assisted-living facility? .... ☐ yes ☒ no
    If **yes**, give us the name and address of the facility, and the amount of the deposit, and answer the following questions.

Name of facility	Address of facility	Amount
		$

    a. Does the facility still have the deposit? .... ☐ yes ☐ no
    b. Did the facility return the deposit?.. ☐ yes ☐ no
    If **yes**, give us the name and address of the person who got the deposit from the facility.

Name	Address

Tax Returns

▶ Did you or your spouse file U.S. income tax returns in the last two years? .... ☒ yes ☐ no

    If yes, you must **send copies** of these returns. If you did not keep copies of your tax returns for the last two years, **you must send a filled-out and signed Form 4506 to the Internal Revenue Service.** Form 4506 is included as part of the Long-Term-Care Supplement if you need to use it.

I certify, under penalty of perjury, that the information on this form is correct and complete to the best of my knowledge. I understand that this information will be used to decide if I can get or continue to get MassHealth payment of long-term-care services. I also understand that I must give proof of the information given on this form and report any changes in this information within 10 days of the change.

If you are acting on behalf of someone in filling out this form, a MassHealth Eligibility Representative Designation Form must also be filled out and sent back with this form. Your signature on this form as an eligibility representative certifies that the information on this form is correct and complete to the best of your knowledge.

x _Harriet M. Knellson_   JUNE 8, 2003
Signature of applicant/member or eligibility representative   Date

X _____   _____
Signature of applicant's/member's spouse   Date

MassHealth

Commonwealth of Massachusetts
Division of Medical Assistance
www.mass.gov/dma

Please print clearly. Fill out all sections. If you need more space to finish any section on this form, please use a separate sheet of paper, and attach it to this form. If you have questions about filling out this form or about the MassHealth Personal-Care Attendant (PCA) Program, call 617-210-5000 and ask for the MassHealth PCA Program manager.

Last name	First name	MI	Telephone number ( )	Social security number	Date of birth / /	Sex ☐ M ☐ F
Street address			City		State	Zip

List and describe below all your medical and mental-health problems. Include anything that makes it hard for you to do daily living activities, like bathing, eating, toileting, dressing, etc., even if you are not getting treatment for the problem.

1. _____

2. _____

3. _____

Please tell us in the chart below if you need hands-on help from another person to do the following daily living activities. If you check "yes" to any of the items below, tell us how often you need help.

Daily living activity	Do you need hands-on help?	How many times a **day** do you need hands-on help?	How many **days a week** do you need hands-on help?
Mobility (moving from bed to chair, walking, or using approved medical equipment)	☐ yes ☐ no		
Taking medications	☐ yes ☐ no		
Bathing (tub, bed bath, shower, or washing chair) or general grooming (like brushing teeth or combing hair)	☐ yes ☐ no		
Dressing/Undressing	☐ yes ☐ no		
Range-of-motion exercises (exercising joints by moving them)	☐ yes ☐ no		
Eating	☐ yes ☐ no		
Toileting (like getting on or off toilet, wiping yourself, getting clothes off and on, or changing diapers)	☐ yes ☐ no		

PCA-SUPP (Rev. 04/03)

Please go to other side. ▶

Please give us the name(s) and relationship to you of the person(s) who now helps you.	
Caregiver name	Relationship to you (like relative, neighbor, personal-care attendant)
Caregiver name	Relationship to you (like relative, neighbor, personal-care attendant)

I certify, under penalty of perjury, that the information on this form is correct and complete to the best of my knowledge.

If you are acting on behalf of someone in filling out this form, a MassHealth Eligibility Representative Designation Form must also be filled out and sent back with this form. Your signature on this form as an eligibility representative certifies that the information on this form is correct and complete to the best of your knowledge.

X_____   _____
Signature of applicant/member or eligibility representative   Date

MassHealth

MASSHEALTH PERMISSION TO SHARE INFORMATION FORM

Commonwealth of Massachusetts
Division of Medical Assistance
www.mass.gov/dma

If you want the Division of Medical Assistance to share information about you with another person or organization, please make sure that you fill out all of the numbered sections below to tell us whom to share your information with and what information you want us to share. If you leave ANY sections blank, your permission will not be valid, and the Division of Medical Assistance will not be able to share your information with the person or organization you listed on this form.

SECTION I

Permission is given for the Division of Medical Assistance and its representatives to share information listed in SECTION II about

_____ with the person or organization listed in SECTION III.

(name of MassHealth applicant or member)

SECTION II

The Division of Medical Assistance may share this information. (Check all that apply.)

☐ Eligibility notices and information about eligibility for and access to MassHealth benefits
☐ Status and notices about disability determination

☐ Other: (please be specific) _____

By giving the Division of Medical Assistance permission to share the information listed above, I am specifically giving permission to share any information about drug and alcohol treatment that is included in that information.
　　☐ Yes, I am giving permission.　☐ No, I am not giving permission.

SECTION III

The Division of Medical Assistance may share the information listed in SECTION II with this person or organization:

Name of person or organization:
Street address:
City, state, zip:
Telephone number: (   )

SECTION IV

The Division of Medical Assistance may share the information listed in SECTION II for the following reasons: (Please note: If you do not want to list reasons, you may simply write: "at my request.")

SECTION V

This permission to share information is good until _____

SECTION VI

I understand that:

♦ the person or organization listed in SECTION III may be able to further share the information that the Division of Medical Assistance gives them. If they do, federal and state privacy laws may not protect the information;

♦ I may cancel this permission at any time by sending a letter to:

> Division of Medical Assistance
> Privacy and Security Office
> 600 Washington Street
> Boston, MA 02111;

♦ the Division of Medical Assistance cannot take back any information that it shared when it had my permission to do so;

♦ if I do not give the Division of Medical Assistance permission to share information, or if I cancel my permission to share information with the person or organization listed in SECTION III, MassHealth benefits will not be affected in any way; and

♦ in certain circumstances, the Division of Medical Assistance may not honor my request to share information.

Signature of applicant/member:	Date:
Print name of applicant/member:	
Applicant/Member SSN:	Applicant/Member date of birth:

(Please Note: The applicant's or member's SSN is required if one has been issued, unless he or she is only applying for or getting MassHealth Limited or Children's Medical Security Plan (CMSP) benefits.)

Print name of person filling out this form:	
Signature of person filling out this form:	Date:
Authority of person filling out this form to act on behalf of the applicant/member:	

♺

MassHealth
Commonwealth of Massachusetts
Division of Medical Assistance
www.mass.gov/dma

MASSHEALTH ELIGIBILITY REPRESENTATIVE DESIGNATION FORM

What an eligibility representative does

You may choose an eligibility representative to help you with some or all of the responsibilities of applying for or getting MassHealth. This person must know enough about you to take responsibility for the correctness of the statements made during the eligibility process. An eligibility representative may fill out an application or review form and other MassHealth eligibility forms, give the Division of Medical Assistance (Division) proof of information given on applications, review forms, and other MassHealth forms, report changes in your income, address, or other circumstances, and get copies of all MassHealth eligibility notices sent to you.

Under 130 CMR 516.007, the Division is allowed to send a copy of all applicant and member eligibility notices to the applicant's or member's institution where he or she is living, and to his or her spouse who is living at home without an Eligibility Representative Designation Form being filled out.

Who can be an eligibility representative

An eligibility representative can be a friend, family member, relative, or other person who has a concern for your well-being and who agrees to help you. An eligibility representative is a person you choose. The Division will not choose an eligibility representative for you. You must designate in writing on this form (please fill out Section I, Part A) whom you want to be your eligibility representative. Your eligibility representative must also fill out Section I, Part B. If at some later time you no longer want this person to be your eligibility representative, you must send a letter stating this to: Division of Medical Assistance, Privacy and Security Office, 600 Washington Street, Boston, MA 02111.

If, because of a mental or physical condition, you cannot designate in writing whom you want to be your eligibility representative, a person who is acting responsibly on your behalf can be your eligibility representative if that person certifies by filling out Section II that you are not able to provide a written designation, and that he or she is acting responsibly on your behalf.

An eligibility representative can also be someone who has been appointed by law to act on your behalf or on behalf of your estate. This person must fill out Section III, and either you or this person must submit to the Division a copy of the applicable legal document stating that this person is lawfully representing you or your estate. This person may be a legal guardian, conservator, holder of power of attorney, or health-care proxy, or, if the applicant or member has died, the estate's administrator or executor.

Please Note: The applicant's or member's SSN is required if one has been issued, unless he or she is only applying for or getting MassHealth Limited or Children's Medical Security Plan (CMSP) benefits.

FRD (04/03)

SECTION I: Eligibility Representative Designation (If applicant or member is able to sign)

I certify that I have chosen the following person to be my eligibility representative, and that I understand the duties and responsibilities this person will have (as explained on the other side of this form).

Eligibility representative name:	

Eligibility representative address:	

Eligibility representative telephone no.: ( )	Relationship to you:

My name:	My SSN:	My date of birth:

My signature:	Date:

I certify that I know enough about the above applicant or member to take responsibility for the correctness of the statements made during the eligibility process, and that I understand my duties and responsibilities as this person's eligibility representative (as explained on the other side of this form).

Eligibility representative signature:	Date:

SECTION II: Eligibility Representative Designation (If applicant or member cannot provide written designation)

I certify that I know enough about the applicant or member named below to take responsibility for the correctness of the statements made during the eligibility process, that I understand my duties and responsibilities as this person's eligibility representative (as explained on the other side of this form), and that this person cannot provide written designation. When necessary and/or possible, I have told this person that the Division will send me a copy of all MassHealth eligibility notices and that this person agrees to this. When necessary and/or possible, I have also told this person that he or she may remove me as eligibility representative at any time by sending a letter to: Division of Medical Assistance, Privacy and Security Office, 600 Washington Street, Boston, MA, 02111.

Eligibility representative name:	

Eligibility representative address:	

Eligibility representative telephone no.: ( )	

Eligibility representative signature:	Date:

Applicant/Member name:	Applicant/Member date of birth:

Applicant/Member SSN:	Your relationship to applicant or member:

SECTION III: Eligibility Representative Designation (appointed by law)

Applicant/Member name:	

Applicant/Member SSN:	Applicant/Member date of birth:

Eligibility representative name:	

Eligibility representative address:	

Eligibility representative telephone no.: ( )	

Eligibility representative signature:	Date:

8-B

REVERE OFFICE
300 OCEAN AVENUE, SUITE 4000
REVERE MA 02151-3675

Commonwealth of Massachusetts
Executive Office of Health
and Human Services
Division of Medical Assistance

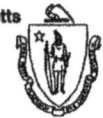

IMPORTANT NOTICE - READ CAREFULLY

REGION	MEC	CAT.	TEL.	SSN	CAN.
			(800)322-1448	3	314
06	550	S			

09/04/2003

MA 02471   FOR:

AS YOU HAVE REQUESTED, THE DIVISION HAS ASSESSED THE VALUE OF YOUR
TOTAL COUNTABLE ASSETS AS OF THE DATE YOU ENTERED THE INSTITUTION,
AND HAS DETERMINED THAT IF YOU REMAIN IN A MEDICAL INSTITUTION AND
APPLY FOR MASSHEALTH, YOUR SPOUSE AT HOME WILL BE ABLE TO KEEP $90660.00
FROM YOUR TOTAL COUNTABLE ASSETS.

THIS AMOUNT WILL BELONG TO YOUR SPOUSE AT HOME AND WILL NOT BE
CONSIDERED IN DETERMINING YOUR ELIGIBILITY FOR MASSHEALTH. A RECIPIENT
OF MASSHEALTH IS ALLOWED TO HAVE $2000 IN ASSETS. YOU WILL MEET THE
ASSET STANDARD FOR MASSHEALTH ELIGIBILITY WHEN YOUR TOTAL COMBINED ASSETS
ARE $92660.00. SINCE THIS AMOUNT IS SUBJECT TO A COST OF LIVING
ADJUSTMENT, YOU SHOULD APPLY FOR MEDICAID WHEN YOUR TOTAL COMBINED
ASSETS ARE WITHIN $5000 OF THE ASSET STANDARD.

A PENALTY WILL BE IMPOSED IF YOU TRANSFER YOUR COUNTABLE ASSETS
FOR LESS THAN THEIR FAIR MARKET VALUE.

PLEASE KEEP THIS NOTICE UNTIL YOU APPLY FOR MASSHEALTH. IF YOU APPLIED
FOR MASSHEALTH AT THE SAME TIME YOU ASKED FOR THIS ASSET ASSESSMENT, YOU
WILL RECEIVE A SEPARATE NOTICE ABOUT YOUR MASSHEALTH ELIGIBILITY.

YOUR SPOUSE MAY HAVE THE RIGHT TO RETAIN A LARGER SHARE OF THE COMBINED
SPOUSAL ASSETS THAN THE AMOUNT INDICATED ABOVE, DEPENDING ON HIS OR HER
MONTHLY INCOME AND MONTHLY NEEDS. THIS INFORMATION REGARDING THE RIGHT
OF THE COMMUNITY SPOUSE TO THE SPOUSAL ASSETS WILL BE PROVIDED AT THE
TIME THAT THE MASSHEALTH ELIGIBILITY OF THE INSTITUTIONALIZED SPOUSE IS
DETERMINED. THIS DETERMINATION WILL BE MADE IN ACCORDANCE WITH DIVISION
REGULATIONS 130 CMR 520.017.

AT THE TIME YOU APPLY FOR MASSHEALTH, IF YOU AND YOUR SPOUSE DISAGREE WITH
THIS DECISION YOU HAVE THE RIGHT TO A FAIR HEARING CONCERNING:
 . THE OWNERSHIP OR AVAILABILITY OF INCOME OR ASSETS
 . THE DETERMINATION OF THE COMMUNITY SPOUSE MONTHLY INCOME
ALLOWANCE OR ASSET ALLOWANCE

YOU MUST REQUEST A FAIR HEARING WITHIN THIRTY DAYS OF YOUR NOTICE
REGARDING MASSHEALTH ELIGIBILITY. THE DIVISION MUST MAKE A FAIR HEARING
DECISION WITHIN NINETY DAYS OF YOUR REQUEST.

THIS NOTICE CONTAINS INFORMATION PURSUANT TO MASSACHUSETTS GENERAL LAWS
CHAPTER 118E, SEC 21A.

YOU MAY WISH TO CONTACT A LOCAL LEGAL SERVICE OFFICE OR COMMUNITY
AGENCY. THEY WILL PROVIDE ADVICE OR REPRESENTATION AT NO CHARGE.
INFORMATION ABOUT THESE SERVICES, IF AVAILABLE IN YOUR AREA, CAN BE
OBTAINED BY CONTACTING YOUR MASSHEALTH ENROLLMENT CENTER.

Continued...

-2-

```
HOW WE COUNTED YOUR ASSETS
--------------------------

MA COUNTABLE ASSETS
   LIFE INSURANCE          35600.00
   PNA ACCOUNT                  .00
   AUTO VALUE                   .00
   BANK ACCOUNT            39563.00
   REAL ESTATE VALUE            .00
   OTHER                  109493.00
TOTAL COUNTABLE ASSETS    184656.00    184656.00
AMOUNT OF ASSETS YOU
   MAY KEEP                 2000.00
AMOUNT OF ASSETS YOUR
   SPOUSE MAY KEEP       + 90660.00
                          ---------
TOTAL ASSETS YOU AND
   YOUR SPOUSE MAY KEEP    92660.00  -  92660.00

AMOUNT YOU ARE OVER MA                  ---------
   ASSET LIMIT                          91996.00
```

8-C

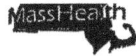

SPOUSAL NOTICE SUPPLEMENT

MassHealth Enrollment Center

367 East St.

Tewksbury, MA 01876

Telephone: (802) 408-1253

Name:_____ Date:_____

Address:_____

Recently your application for MassHealth was denied because you and your spouse have countable assets that are over the MassHealth limits. In accordance with 130 CMR 520.017(A), if your spouse at home (the community spouse) needs extra income to remain in the community, he or she may be allowed to keep a larger share of your combined assets to produce this extra income to bring the community spouse's total income up to a certain level. To find out if the community spouse can keep a larger share of your combined assets, you must ask for a fair hearing, and show that:

- the community spouse's income is less than the Minimum Monthly Maintenance Needs Allowance (described below); and
- the community spouse needs extra assets to produce additional income to remain in the community.

The hearing officer will consider the community spouse's right to keep extra assets before allowing income from the institutionalized spouse to be available to the community spouse.

See the other side of this notice for information about your appeal rights. To ask for a fair hearing, fill out the other side of this notice and send it to the Board of Hearings.

The Division may deduct certain amounts from the institutionalized spouse's countable income in accordance with 130 CMR 520.025. The enclosed worksheet shows the deductions that are allowed based on your current financial circumstances. These deductions are subject to change when your financial circumstances or the federal needs standards change.

<u>Minimum Monthly Maintenance Needs Allowance</u>: MassHealth determines the monthly amount the community spouse needs for his or her living expenses using a standard of need set by federal law, <u>and the</u> actual shelter expenses of the community spouse. This monthly amount is called the Minimum Monthly Maintenance Needs Allowance (MMMNA).

<u>Spousal Maintenance Needs Allowance</u>: When a community spouse's monthly income is less than the MMMNA, MassHealth can allow an amount from the institutionalized spouse's monthly income to meet this need. This amount is called the spousal maintenance needs allowance (SMNA).

<u>Family Maintenance Needs Allowance</u>: The family maintenance needs allowance (FMNA) may be allowed to meet the maintenance needs of certain family members living with the community spouse.

<u>Patient-Paid Amount</u>: When the institutionalized spouse must contribute a monthly amount toward the cost of his or her care, this amount is called the patient-paid amount (PPA). The PPA is based on the institutionalized spouse's income less certain deductions

This notice contains information pursuant to Massachusetts General Laws c. 118E, § 21A.

SNS (Rev. 07/99)

MONTHLY MAINTENANCE NEEDS ALLOWANCE WORKSHEET

Below is an explanation of how the Division determines the monthly income allowance for a spouse or family.

SECTION I: CALCULATION OF THE MINIMUM MONTHLY MAINTENANCE NEEDS ALLOWANCE (MMMNA) FOR THE COMMUNITY SPOUSE

Shelter Expenses for Community Spouse's Principal Place of Residence

Rent or Mortgage	$
Property Taxes and Insurance	$
Required Maintenance Charge for a Condominium or Cooperative	$
Standard Deduction for Utility Expenses*	+ ⟨ *425 Heated* / *258 Unheated*
TOTAL Shelter Expenses	=
Subtract Standard Shelter Expense*	- 455
Excess Shelter Amount	= (Enter zero if total shelter expenses are less than the federal standard maintenance allowance.*)
Add Federal Standard Maintenance Allowance*	+ 1515

MMMNA for Community Spouse
[May not exceed established maximum* except following a fair hearing in accordance with 130 CMR 520.017(D).]   = $

SECTION II: CALCULATION OF THE SPOUSAL MAINTENANCE NEEDS ALLOWANCE (SMNA) FOR THE COMMUNITY SPOUSE

Gross Monthly Income of Community Spouse

Pension(s)	$
Social Security/RSDI Benefits	$
Income from Spousal Assets	$
Other Income (Trust, Earnings, etc.)	+

Subtract TOTAL Gross Income of Community Spouse from MMMNA for Community Spouse (in Section I)   - $

Additional Monthly Income Need of Community Spouse (SMNA)   = $

Note: You may ask for a hearing to keep more assets to generate additional income to meet the MMMNA.

---

*These amounts are established by federal law.

MMNA (07/99)

SECTION III: CALCULATION OF THE FAMILY MAINTENANCE NEEDS ALLOWANCE (FMNA) FOR CERTAIN FAMILY MEMBERS LIVING WITH THE COMMUNITY SPOUSE [Show a separate calculation specific to each family member (excluding the community spouse).]

Federal Standard Maintenance Allowance* $_____

Subtract Gross Monthly Income of Family Member   _____

Divide Difference by 3   ÷3 _____

Monthly Income Need of Family Member Living with the Community Spouse (FMNA)   = $_____

SECTION IV: CALCULATION OF INCOME AND PATIENT-PAID AMOUNT (PPA) OF INSTITUTIONALIZED SPOUSE

Monthly Income of Institutionalized Spouse

Social Security/RSDI Benefits (Net) $_____

Pension(s) (Gross) $_____

Other (Gross)   +_____

TOTAL Income of Institutionalized Spouse   = $_____

Deductions Allowed from Income of Institutionalized Spouse

Personal Needs Allowance (PNA)** $_____

SMNA $_____

FMNA $_____

Health-Care Coverage (other than Medicare) or Other Incurred Expenses   +_____

Subtract TOTAL Deductions from TOTAL Income of Institutionalized Spouse   – $_____

Institutionalized Spouse's PPA   = $_____

*This amount is established by federal law.

**This amount is established by state and federal laws.

8-D

REVERE OFFICE
300 OCEAN AVENUE, SUITE 4000
REVERE MA 02151-3675

and Human Services
Division of Medical Assistance

<To request a hearing, see the other side of this form>

REGION	MEC	CAT.	TEL.	SSN	CAN.
			(800)322-1448	6	308
06	550	5			

12/31/2003

FOR:

THE DIVISION HAS APPROVED
MASSHEALTH BENEFITS FOR THE FOLLOWING PEOPLE:

YOUR ELIGIBILITY BEGINS ON 07/14/2003.

THE DIVISION MAY ALSO PAY FOR MEDICAL SERVICES YOU RECEIVED IN THE
THREE MONTHS BEFORE THE MONTH YOU APPLIED IF YOU WERE ELIGIBLE DURING
THAT TIME. IF YOU HAVE NOT YET APPLIED FOR THESE BENEFITS, CONTACT
YOUR WORKER RIGHT AWAY.

STARTING IN 07/2003, YOU WILL OWE YOUR FACILITY $110.69 EVERY MONTH
TO HELP PAY FOR YOUR CARE. YOUR FACILITY WILL BILL YOU $110.69 EVERY
MONTH. THIS IS CALLED YOUR "PATIENT PAID AMOUNT".

YOU WILL SOON GET A MASSHEALTH CARD. KEEP YOUR MASSHEALTH CARD WITH YOU
AT ALL TIMES AND ALWAYS SHOW IT TO THE PROVIDER BEFORE GETTING MEDICAL
SERVICES.

YOU MUST REPORT ANY CHANGES IN YOUR HEALTH INSURANCE, ADDRESS, INCOME,
FAMILY SIZE, IMMIGRANT STATUS, OR OTHER SITUATION TO YOUR MASSHEALTH EN-
ROLLMENT CENTER WITHIN 10 DAYS. THESE CHANGES MAY AFFECT YOUR ELIGIBILITY.

YOU MAY ALSO GET HELP FROM THE CUSTOMER SERVICE CENTER AT 1-800-841-2900
IF YOU:
. NEED INFORMATION ABOUT YOUR MASSHEALTH COVERED SERVICES; OR
. NEED TRANSPORTATION FOR A MEDICAL APPOINTMENT AND QUALIFY FOR IT.

CALL THE MASSHEALTH ENROLLMENT CENTER AT (800)322-1448 IF YOU HAVE
ANY QUESTIONS ABOUT ELIGIBILITY.

Continued...

Name: SSN: Date: 12/31/2003

Request for a Fair Hearing

Your Right to Appeal: If you disagree with any action or inaction by the Division of Medical Assistance, you have the right to appeal and receive a fair hearing before an impartial hearing officer. The Division must receive your request for a fair hearing no later than 30 days from the date you received the Division's official written notice notifying you of the action to be taken.

How to Appeal: If you wish to request a fair hearing, send this completed form to: **Division of Medical Assistance, Board of Hearings, 2 Boylston Street, Boston, MA 02116 or fax to (617) 210-5820.** Please keep the second copy of this form for your information.

If You Are Currently Receiving Assistance: If the Board of Hearings receives your fair hearing request prior to the implementation date or, if later, within 10 days of the mailing of the notice, your assistance will be continued until a decision is made on your appeal. If you receive assistance during your appeal, but lose your appeal, the Division can recover from you the amount of assistance to which you were not entitled. If you do not wish to continue to receive assistance during your appeal, please check Box A below. If you do not receive assistance during your appeal, and you win your appeal, the Division will promptly restore any loss of assistance benefits for the affected time period.

Date of Fair Hearing: You will be notified by mail at least 10 days before the fair hearing of the date, time, and place so that you will have time to prepare your case. If you wish to have a fair hearing scheduled as soon as possible, check Box B below. If you have good cause of a serious nature for not being able to attend the hearing, you must contact the Board of Hearings at (617) 210-5800 or 1-800-655-0338 at least one week before the hearing date. Failure to reschedule or appear on time at the hearing without documented good cause may result in the dismissal of your appeal.

Your Right to Be Assisted at The Hearing: At the hearing, you may represent yourself or be accompanied by an attorney or representative at your own expense. You may contact a local legal service or community agency to obtain advice or representation at no cost. To obtain information about legal service or community agencies; contact your MassHealth Enrollment Center.

If You Need an Interpreter: If you are not fluent in English and would like an interpreter, the Board of Hearings will provide an interpreter for you. Please write on this appeal request that you need an interpreter or call the Board of Hearings at (617) 210-5800 or 1-800-655-0338 at least one week before the hearing.

Your Right to Review Your Assistance Files: You and/or your representative will be permitted to see your assistance files before the hearing by scheduling an appointment with your eligibility worker in advance of the fair hearing. You or your representative may subpoena witnesses, present evidence, and cross-examine witnesses. The hearing officer must make a decision on all evidence presented at the fair hearing.

NONDISCRIMINATION NOTICE FOR MEMBERS: Under federal and state law the Massachusetts Division of Medical Assistance does not discriminate on the basis of race, color, sex, sexual orientation, national origin, religion, creed, age, or handicap. For help with any matter pertaining to this policy, we encourage you to contact the Board of Hearings at (617) 210-5800 or 1-800-655-0338.

COMPLETE ALL APPROPRIATE SECTIONS - PRINT CLEARLY

Name of Applicant or Member:_____

Address:_____

Telephone No.:( )_____ MassHealth I.D. or SSN:_____

Cardholder's Name on MassHealth card (if different):_____

☐ I request an interpreter (indicate language:_____) to be provided by the Board of Hearings.

Signature:_____ Date:_____

My appeal representative is:_____ Title:_____

Address:_____

Telephone No.:( )_____

I,_____, hereby request a fair hearing before a hearing officer of the Board of Hearings. The reason I wish to request a fair hearing is:_____

☐ A. I do not wish to continue receiving assistance during the appeal process.

☐ B. I request an expedited hearing because:_____

```
HOW WE DETERMINED YOUR
-----------------------
    MONTHLY PATIENT PAID AMOUNT (PPA)
    ---------------------------------

UNEARNED INCOME
    SOCIAL SECURITY/RRB        843.00
    COUNTABLE VETERANS'
        BENEFITS                 .00
    OTHER                     161.69
TOTAL UNEARNED INCOME                   1004.69   1004.69

COUNTABLE EARNED INCOME                     .00 +     .00
                                               --------
TOTAL COUNTABLE INCOME                            1004.69

OTHER ALLOWANCES
    PERSONAL NEEDS ALLOW        60.00
    AMT TO MAINTAIN HOME       749.00
    SPOUSE IN HOME               .00
    FAMILY MEMBERS IN HOME       .00
    HEALTH INSURANCE           85.00
    OTHER MEDICAL               .00
TOTAL ALLOWANCES               894.00           -  894.00
                                                  --------

NET COUNTABLE INCOME                               110.69

AMOUNT YOU PAY NURSING FACILITY (PPA)              110.69
```

RA- NO. 13

Name: .   SSN: Date: 12/31/2003

Request for a Fair Hearing

Your Right to Appeal: If you disagree with any action or inaction by the Division of Medical Assistance, you have the right to appeal and receive a fair hearing before an impartial hearing officer. The Division must receive your request for a fair hearing no later than <u>30 days</u> from the date you received the Division's official written notice notifying you of the action to be taken.

How to Appeal: If you wish to request a fair hearing, send this completed form to: **Division of Medical Assistance, Board of Hearings, 2 Boylston Street, Boston, MA 02116** or fax to **(617) 210-5820**. Please keep the second copy of this form for your information.

If You Are Currently Receiving Assistance: If the Board of Hearings receives your fair hearing request prior to the implementation date or, if later, within 10 days of the mailing of the notice, your assistance will be continued until a decision is made on your appeal. If you receive assistance during your appeal, but lose your appeal, the Division can recover from you the amount of assistance to which you were not entitled. If you do not wish to continue to receive assistance during your appeal, please check Box A below. If you do not receive assistance during your appeal, and you win your appeal, the Division will promptly restore any loss of assistance benefits for the affected time period.

Date of Fair Hearing: You will be notified by mail at least <u>10 days</u> before the fair hearing of the <u>date, time, and place</u> so that you will have time to prepare your case. If you wish to have a fair hearing scheduled as soon as possible, check Box B below. If you have good cause of a serious nature for not being able to attend the hearing, you must contact the Board of Hearings at **(617) 210-5800 or 1-800-655-0338** at least one week before the hearing date. Failure to reschedule or appear on time at the hearing without documented good cause may result in the dismissal of your appeal.

Your Right to Be Assisted at The Hearing: At the hearing, you may represent yourself or be accompanied by an attorney or representative at your own expense. You may contact a local legal service or community agency to obtain advice or representation at no cost. To obtain information about legal service or community agencies, contact your MassHealth Enrollment Center.

If You Need an Interpreter: If you are not fluent in English and would like an interpreter, the Board of Hearings will provide an interpreter for you. Please write on this appeal request that you need an interpreter or call the Board of Hearings at **(617) 210-5800 or 1-800-655-0338** at least one week before the hearing.

Your Right to Review Your Assistance Files: You and/or your representative will be permitted to see your assistance files before the hearing by scheduling an appointment with your eligibility worker in advance of the fair hearing. You or your representative may subpoena witnesses, present evidence, and cross-examine witnesses. The hearing officer must make a decision on all evidence presented at the fair hearing.

NONDISCRIMINATION NOTICE FOR MEMBERS: Under federal and state law the Massachusetts Division of Medical Assistance does not discriminate on the basis of race, color, sex, sexual orientation, national origin, religion, creed, age, or handicap. For help with any matter pertaining to this policy, we encourage you to contact the Board of Hearings at (617) 210-5800 or 1-800-655-0338.

COMPLETE ALL APPROPRIATE SECTIONS - PRINT CLEARLY

Name of Applicant or Member:_____

Address:_____

Telephone No.:(   )_____ MassHealth I.D. or SSN:_____

Cardholder's Name on MassHealth card (if different):_____

☐ I request an interpreter (indicate language:_____) to be provided by the Board of Hearings.

Signature:_____ Date:_____

My appeal representative is:_____ Title:_____

Address:_____

Telephone No.:(   )_____

I,_____, hereby request a fair hearing before a hearing officer of the Board of Hearings. The reason I wish to request a fair hearing is:_____

_____

☐ A. I do not wish to continue receiving assistance during the appeal process.

☐ B. I request an expedited hearing because:_____

_____

8-E

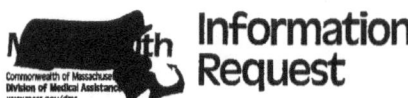

Information Request

Commonwealth of Massachusetts
Division of Medical Assistance
www.mass.gov/dma

Date:

MassHealth Enrollment Center	
Address:	300 Ocean Avenue, Suite 4000
City/Town/Zip:	Revere, MA 02151
MassHealth worker:	
Telephone:	1-800-322-1448 Ext.: 577
TTY:	1-877-668-4499 (for the deaf and hard of hearing)
Fax:	781-485-3400

You must send copies of the information checked off on this form by **09/21/03** to the MassHealth Enrollment Center listed above. (Please put your name and social security number on the information you are sending to us and attach this request form.)

If you do not give us the information we are asking for, your MassHealth benefits may be denied or stopped. If you need help to get any information, call your MassHealth worker at the telephone number listed above.

Applicant/Member name

Applicant/Member Social Security Number

☑ First Request   ☐ Second Request

Basic Information

☐ **Immigration Status**: a copy of both sides of **all** immigration cards or other documents that show your immigration status

☑ **Health Insurance**: a copy of both sides of **all** health insurance cards and a copy of your current premium bill

☐ **Third-Party Liability** (enclosed): fill out and send back the Assignment of Third-Party-Recovery packet.

☐ **MassHealth Disability Supplement** (enclosed): fill out, date, sign, and send back. Be sure to sign all medical release forms.

☐ **Spousal and Family Supplement** (enclosed): fill out, date, sign, and send back. Be sure to give us proof of information.

Long-Term-Care Information

(You must make sure the facility gives us this information.)

☑ **Residence**: notification of admission to facility (SC-1)

☑ **Private Payment for Long-Term-Care Services**: statement from facility showing amount paid to date and dates of coverage

☑ **Nursing Facility Screening Notification**

☑ **Personal Needs Account**: personal needs account statement from facility showing activity within the last 45 days

Assets Information

☑ **Tax Returns**: a copy of your federal tax returns for the last two years for both you and your spouse. If not available, send a filled-out and signed Form 4506 (enclosed with this form) to the Internal Revenue Service and send a copy to your MassHealth worker.

☑ **Bank Accounts** (including accounts set up for burial only):

    1. Provide bank statements from 07/01/02 to 06/17/03 for acct #   **. Also verify all deposits and withdrawals over $1000.00 from 07/01/02 to present.**

☐ **Life Insurance**: a copy of the first page of all life-insurance policies, including life insurance policies set up for burial only. If total face value of all policies exceeds $1,500, also send a letter from the insurance company showing the current cash-surrender value (for all policies except term policies).

MIR-R-0 (Rev. 08/02)

continued on back ▶

Assets Information *continued*

✓ ☑ **Trust:** all trust documents and accountings that show all assets in the trust including current balance and all activity during the period from **07/01/02** to **07/31/03** Also send proof of all income distributed during this period, a schedule of trust assets, and a schedule of beneficiaries. If a realty trust, send a copy of deed.

☐ **Burial Plan:** prepaid and dated irrevocable contract or irrevocable trust signed by both you and the funeral home director, or if unavailable an itemized statement from the funeral home director to prove the existence of an irrevocable burial contract or irrevocable trust, an irrevocable trust instrument, any burial insurance policy, or any statement signed by you designating a burial account or life insurance policy for burial expenses

☐ **Real Estate:** a copy of the deed(s) and current tax bill for all properties that you and/or your spouse have a legal interest in. Also send the following:

　☐ Birth certificate proving relationship of child, sibling, or dependent relative
　☐ Medical financial-need statement for dependent relative
　☐ Statement of Expectation to Return Home (enclosed): filled out and signed by a doctor
　☐ Medical statement for disabled/blind child
　☐ Medical statement for son or daughter who provided care to you for the past two years
　☐ Document showing duration of relative's residence in home of institutionalized individual

☐ **Long-Term-Care Insurance:** all long-term-care insurance policies

☐ **Vehicles/Mobile Homes:** titles or registrations to all vehicles and loan agreements; bill of sale for mobile homes

☐ **Stocks/Bonds/Other:** copies of certificates, current quote from stockholder, daily paper, or investment firm to prove current value, copies of savings bonds, and financial statements showing activity during the 36-month period from _____ to _____

☐ **Annuity:** contract showing owner's name, name of person getting income, company name, dates of purchase, purchase price, and amount of income received

☐ **Transferred Resources:** all documents that transfer assets or income, showing the date of transfer, value of asset or income on date of transfer, and name of person to whom transfer was made

☐ **Asset Assessment:** proof of all assets owned by you and/or your spouse on the date of admission to the medical institution. You must send copies of the following information:

Income Information

☑ **General Income:** proof of all income showing gross amounts and deductions, like two current pay stubs, federal tax returns, pension stub showing gross amount, or other proofs of income and business expenses for the past 12 months

☑ **Rental Income:** for all units, proof of rental income and expenses for the past 12 months, including taxes, mortgage statement, insurance, heat and water if provided, and repairs and maintenance

☐ **Spousal Income and Expenses:** proof of all gross income received and all living expenses, like rent, mortgage, taxes, insurance, condominium fees, heat, and utilities

Other Information

☑ 1. Please fill out enclosed forms ERD section III completley, and all sections of PSI completely.

☐
☐
☐
☐

8-F

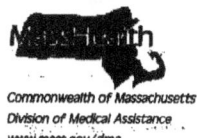

Commonwealth of Massachusetts
Division of Medical Assistance
www.mass.gov/dma

MassHealth Enrollment Center
300 Ocean Avenue, Suite 4000
Revere, MA 02151
Date:

MassHealth Denial Notice

Re: Applicant name   SSN

We have reviewed your application for MassHealth. You are not eligible for MassHealth because:

you did not send in the current medex bill, 1/03 thru 12/03 on all accounts including Eastern no. 402611388, and complete page 5 of the application listing all bank accounts

Regulation Cite: 130 CMR 515.008, 520.007, 517.008

If your application for MassHealth was denied because you did not give us the information or proof we needed to decide if you are eligible for MassHealth, you can either:

- send us some of the needed information or proof within 30 days of the date on this notice (This means that if you are eligible for MassHealth, the date we get the needed information or proof will be your reapplication date.); or

- ask for a fair hearing if you want us to go back to your original application date.

You have the right to apply for MassHealth at any time.

If you think our decision is wrong, you have the right to ask for a fair hearing. To ask for a fair hearing, read and fill out the other side of this notice. Keep the second copy of this notice for your information.

_____
MassHealth Enrollment Center Representative

1 800 322 1448 Ext. 588
1 877 668 4499 TTY
(for the deaf and hard of hearing)

Cc:

NFL-5-R-0 (Rev. 08/02)   Page 1 of 2

Your Right to Appeal: If you disagree with any action or inaction by the Division of Medical Assistance, you have the right to appeal and receive a fair hearing before an impartial hearing officer. The Division must receive your request for a fair hearing no later than 30 days from the date you received the Division's official written notice notifying you of the action to be taken.

How to Appeal: If you wish to request a fair hearing, send this completed form to: Division of Medical Assistance, Board of Hearings, 2 Boylston Street, Boston, MA 02116 or fax to 617-210-5820. Please keep the second copy of this form for your information.

If You Are Currently Receiving Assistance: If the Board of Hearings receives your fair hearing request within 10 days from the mailing date of the Division's written notice to you, your assistance will be continued until a decision is made on your appeal. If you receive assistance during your appeal, but lose your appeal, the Division can recover from you the amount of assistance to which you were not entitled. If you do not wish to continue to receive assistance during your appeal, please check Box A below. If you do not receive assistance during your appeal, and you win your appeal, the Division will promptly restore any loss of assistance benefits for the affected time period.

Date of Fair Hearing: You will be notified by mail at least 10 days before the fair hearing of the date, time, and place so that you will have time to prepare your case. If you wish to have a fair hearing scheduled as soon as possible, check Box B below. If you have good cause of a serious nature for not being able to attend the hearing, you must contact the Board of Hearings at 617-210-5800 or 1-800-655-0338 at least one week before the hearing date. Failure to reschedule or appear on time at the hearing without documented good cause may result in the dismissal of your appeal.

Your Right to Be Assisted at the Hearing: At the hearing, you may represent yourself or be accompanied by an attorney or representative at your own expense. You may contact a local legal service or community agency to obtain advice or representation at no cost. To obtain information about legal service or community agencies, contact your MassHealth Enrollment Center.

If You Need an Interpreter: If you are not fluent in English and would like an interpreter, the Board of Hearings will provide an interpreter for you. Please write on this appeal request that you need an interpreter or call the Board of Hearings at 617-210-5800 or 1-800-655-0338 at least one week before the hearing.

Your Right to Review Your Assistance Files: You and/or your representative will be permitted to see your assistance files before the hearing by scheduling an appointment with your eligibility worker in advance of the fair hearing. You or your representative may subpoena witnesses, present evidence, and cross-examine witnesses. The hearing officer must make a decision on all evidence presented at the fair hearing.

NONDISCRIMINATION NOTICE FOR MEMBERS: Under federal and state law the Massachusetts Division of Medical Assistance does not discriminate on the basis of race, color, sex, sexual orientation, national origin, religion, creed, age, or handicap. For help with any matter pertaining to this policy, we encourage you to contact the Board of Hearings at 617-210-5800 or 1-800-655-0338.

Request for a Fair Hearing

COMPLETE ALL APPROPRIATE SECTIONS - PRINT CLEARLY

NAME OF APPLICANT OR MEMBER:

ADDRESS:

TELEPHONE NO.: (   )

MASSHEALTH I.D. OR SSN:

CARDHOLDER'S NAME ON MASSHEALTH CARD (IF DIFFERENT):

☐ I REQUEST AN INTERPRETER

INDICATE LANGUAGE:

TO BE PROVIDED BY THE BOARD OF HEARINGS.

SIGNATURE:

DATE:

MY AUTHORIZED REPRESENTATIVE IS:

TITLE:

ADDRESS:

TELEPHONE NO.: (   )

I, _____ HEREBY REQUEST A FAIR HEARING BEFORE A HEARING OFFICER OF THE BOARD OF HEARINGS. THE REASON I WISH TO REQUEST A FAIR HEARING IS:

☐ A. I DO NOT WISH TO CONTINUE RECEIVING ASSISTANCE DURING THE APPEAL PROCESS.

☐ B. I REQUEST AN EXPEDITED HEARING BECAUSE:

MA/RFH/M (Rev. 08/97)

8-G

REQUEST FOR A FAIR HEARING

Your Right to Appeal: If you disagree with any action or inaction taken by the Division of Medical Assistance, you have the right to appeal and receive a fair hearing before an impartial hearing officer. The Division must receive your request for a fair hearing no later than *30 days* from the date you received the Division's official written notice notifying you of the action to be taken.

How to Appeal: If you wish to request a fair hearing, send this completed form to: **Division of Medical Assistance, Board of Hearings, 2 Boylston Street, Boston, MA 02116 or fax to (617) 210-5820.** Please keep the second copy of this form for your information.

If You are Currently Receiving Assistance: If the board of hearing receives your fair hearing request within *10 days* from the mailing date of the Division's written notice to you, your assistance will be continued until a decision is made on your appeal. If you receive assistance during your appeal, but lose your appeal, the Division can recover from you the amount of assistance to which you were not entitled. If you do not wish to continue to receive assistance during your appeal, please check Box A below. If you do not receive assistance during your appeal, and you win your appeal, the Division will promptly restore any loss of assistance benefits for the affected time period.

Date of Fair Hearing: You will be notified by mail at least *10 days* before the fair hearing of the *date, time and place* so that you will have time to prepare your case. If you wish to have a fair hearing scheduled as soon as possible, check Box B below. If you have a good cause of a serious nature for not being able to attend the hearing, you must contact the Board of Hearings at *(617) 210-5800 or 1-800-655-0338* at least one week before the hearing date. Failure to reschedule or appear on time at the hearing without documented good cause may result in the dismissal of your appeal.

Your Right to Be Assisted At the Hearing: At the hearing, you may represent yourself or be accompanied by an attorney or representative at your own expense. You may contact a local legal service or community agency to obtain advice or representation at no cost. To obtain information about legal service or community agencies, contact your Medical Assistance office.

If You Need an Interpreter: If you are not fluent in English and would like an interpreter, the Board of Hearings will provide an interpreter for you. Please write on this appeal request that you need an interpreter or call the Board of Hearings at *(617) 210-5800 or 1-800-655-0338* at least one week before the hearing.

Your Right to Review Your Assistance Files: You and/or your representative will be permitted to see your assistance files before the hearing by scheduling an appointment with your eligibility worker in advance of the fair hearing. You or your representative may subpoena witnesses, present evidence, and cross-examine witnesses. The hearing officer must make a decision on all evidence presented at the fair hearing.

Non Discrimination Notice For Recipients: Under federal and state law the Massachusetts Division of Medical Assistance does not discriminate on the basis of race, color, sex, sexual orientation, national origin, religion, creed, age, or handicap. For help with any matter pertaining to this policy, we encourage you to contact the Board of Hearings at *(617) 210-5800 or 1-800-655-0338.*

Complete All Appropriate Sections-Print Clearly

Name of Applicant or Recipient: _____

Address: _____

Telephone No.: _____ Medical Assistance ID or SSN: _____

Cardholder's Name on MassHealth card (if different): _____

I request an interpreter (indicate language _____) to be provided by the Board of Hearings.

Signature: _____ Date: _____

My authorized Representative is: _____ Title: _____

Address: _____ Telephone No.: _____

I, _____ , hereby request a fair hearing before a hearing officer at the Board of Hearings. The reason I wish to request a fair hearing is: _____

_____

_____

☐ A. I do not wish to receive assistance during the appeal process.

☐ B. I request an expedited hearing because: _____

_____

8-H

DMA BOARD OF APPEALS

Memorandum

To: Hearing Officer, D.M.A.

Subj: Institutionalized spouse (IS):

(Nursing Home)

Community Spouse (CS):

Revised Community Spouse Resource Allowance

Introduction

The Appellant CS,   , filed a long term care Medicaid application on behalf of her husband, the IS,   , on or about   , 2003, at the Tewksbury MassHealth Enrollment Center.

By notice dated   , 2003, the DMA made a determination that the couple had spousal assets valued at $ and attributed $, to the Community Spouse (CS), and the balance, $ to the nursing home spouse (IS). The application was denied because of the excess assets attributed to the IS.

This matter is on appeal from that   , 2003, denial of Medicaid eligibility for the IS. His wife has requested that the   2003, assessment of assets, be reviewed at the hearing, that a revised community spouse resource allowance be made at the same time, and, further, that a determination be made that the community spouse is entitled to a community spouse monthly income allowance (CSMIA), all pursuant to the provisions of 130 CMR 520.017 and G.L. c. 118E § 21A.

Facts

The IS was admitted as a resident at the   Nursing Home in   , MA, on   , where he remains.

The CS occupies their home at   , MA. She pays the following monthly shelter costs: real estate taxes ($); homeowners' insurance ($), and pays all utilities. As of the date of her husband's admission to the nursing home, she had, and continues to have, monthly shelter expenses of $ and pays

all utilities, including her telephone, and is thus entitled to a utility allowance of $
. The total of these figures,   , is relevant in the determination of her Minimum
Monthly Maintenance Needs Allowance (MMMNA). Her only income was a
monthly Social Security check in the amount of $. As of the operative date
(the   , 2003, admission), the couple owned countable assets that totaled $
in value.

Community spouse's MMMNA

The first step in determining the eligibility for a revised CSRA is to determine
the CS's Minimum Monthly Maintenance Needs Allowance (MMMNA). To do
so, her shelter costs are computed to determine whether they exceed 30% of the
basic allowance of $1,515.00. In this case, the shelter costs total $ which
exceeds the 30% figure of $455.00 by $. Her MMMNA, then, is the basic
allowance, $1,515.00, plus the shelter differential of $, for a total of $.
Her income is her monthly Social Security pension of $. In order to meet
her MMMNA, she needs to retain sufficient resources to generate the difference:
$. Her share of the spousal assets ($) generate income of $
per month (the highest rate quoted in the Bank Rate Monitor Index is   %).
Up until September 1, 2003, the CS would have been entitled to retain sufficient
spousal assets beyond her basic asset allowance in order to generate the shortfall.

With advent of the so-called "income first" rule, however, [130 C.M.R.
520.017(C)(2)], the hearing officer must first look to the IS's income to determine
whether he has monthly income which may be imputed to the CS in order for her
to be able to meet her MMMNA. The IS's monthly income consists of Social
Security ($) and $. We contend that the hearing officer, in the process of determining the CS's revised CSRA, is foreclosed by federal law
from imputing the IS's Social Security benefits to the CS. Federal statutory law, at
42 U.S.C. § 407 (attached as Exhibit A), prohibits the involuntary assignment or
alienation of Social Security benefits, which shall not "be subject to execution, levy,
attachment, garnishment or other legal process". In the case of *Robbins v. DeBuono*,
(text of opinion attached as Exhibit B), the U.S. 2nd Circuit Court of appeals held
that "legal process" includes the Medicaid program's proceedings to determine the
CS's assets allowance (and the IS's eligibility of Medicaid coverage) and therefore
would violate the anti-alienation provisions of 42 U.S.C. § 407, where the IS's Social
Security benefits were imputed to the CS.

The IS's income consists of the following:

Social Security benefits: $

Other (   ): $

Only $ of the IS's income may be lawfully imputed to the CS, in the determination of her revised CSRA:

CS's MMMNA

CS's SS and pension income:

Income from her share of marital assets:

Permissible imputed income from IS:

CS's total income:

Since the CS's total income remains below the MMMNA by $, she should be allowed to retain additional marital assets to generate the difference at 2.2%. Her revised CSRA should be $ (or the total of marital assets).

In addition, where the income from all sources remains below the CS's MMMNA, she is entitled to a Community Spouse Monthly Income Allowance in the amount of $ so that her income will meet her MMMNA. 130 C.M.R. 510.017(C)(3).

CSRA policy: 130 CMR 520.017

Under current regulations, 130 CMR 520.017, the CS is entitled to retain all spousal assets owned as of the assessment date, and to a community spouse monthly income allowance of $ from her husband's income. The conclusion is based on the facts outlined above.

Conclusion

Accordingly, the CS should be allowed to retain all of the spousal assets in order to generate sufficient income to bring her monthly income up to the MMMNA. The shortfall after the income from all marital assets is imputed to her should result in a monthly spousal income allowance of $ in order to bring her income up to meet her MMMNA.

Respectfully submitted,

_____

8-I

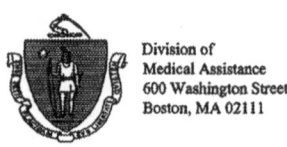

Division of
Medical Assistance
600 Washington Street
Boston, MA 02111

Name:
Social Security Number:
Date:

This notice is sent in response to your request to have the Division of Medical Assistance pay for nursing facility services. In order for the Division to pay for nursing facility services, you must be both clinically and financially eligible for services. This notice is about your clinical eligibility. You will receive a seperate notice about your financial eligibility.

The Division's screenings to determine clinical eligibility for nursing facility services are conducted by <u>North Shore Elder Services</u>, Aging Services Access Point (ASAP). The ASAP nurse reviewed your case in accordance with the Division's regulations at130 CMR 456.408 and has determined:

☐ You **are** clinically eligible for nursing facility services for up to 90 days. If you are not discharged, your continued eligibility is subject to review prior to the 90th day.

☒ You **are** clinically eligible for nursing facility services for more than 90 days. Your continued eligibility is subject to periodic review.

☐ You **are not** eligible for nursing facility services because:

☐ Your medical need is less than required for the Division to pay for nursing facility services.

☐ Your medical needs can be met in the community and services are available.

You have the right to appeal this decision. See attachment.

Official Use Only	
Code: 3E	_____, R.N.
Date: Date of Financial Eligibility	North Shore Elder Services 152 Sylvan Street Danvers MA 01923 (978) 750-4540

ASAP NFCONV-O (Rev. 07/99)

REQUEST FOR A FAIR HEARING

Your Right to Appeal: If you disagree with any action or inaction taken by the Division of Medical Assistance, you have the right to appeal and receive a fair hearing before an impartial hearing officer. The Division must receive your request for a fair hearing no later than *30 days* from the date you received the Division's official written notice notifying you of the action to be taken.

How to Appeal: If you wish to request a fair hearing, send this completed form to: **Division of Medical Assistance, Board of Hearings, 2 Boylston Street, Boston, MA 02116 or fax to (617) 210-5820.** Please keep the second copy of this form for your information.

If You are Currently Receiving Assistance: If the board of hearing receives your fair hearing request within *10 days* from the mailing date of the Division's written notice to you, your assistance will be continued until a decision is made on your appeal. If you receive assistance during your appeal, but lose your appeal, the Division can recover from you the amount of assistance to which you were not entitled. If you do not wish to continue to receive assistance during your appeal, please check Box A below. If you do not receive assistance during your appeal, and you win your appeal, the Division will promptly restore any loss of assistance benefits for the affected time period.

Date of Fair Hearing: You will be notified by mail at least *10 days* before the fair hearing of the *date, time and place* so that you will have time to prepare your case. If you wish to have a fair hearing scheduled as soon as possible, check Box B below. If you have a good cause of a serious nature for not being able to attend the hearing, you must contact the Board of Hearings at *(617) 210-5800 or 1-800-655-0338* at least one week before the hearing date. Failure to reschedule or appear on time at the hearing without documented good cause may result in the dismissal of your appeal.

Your Right to Be Assisted At the Hearing: At the hearing, you may represent yourself or be accompanied by an attorney or representative at your own expense. You may contact a local legal service or community agency to obtain advice or representation at no cost. To obtain information about legal service or community agencies, contact your Medical Assistance office.

If You Need an Interpreter: If you are not fluent in English and would like an interpreter, the Board of Hearings will provide an interpreter for you. Please write on this appeal request that you need an interpreter or call the Board of Hearings at *(617) 210-5800 or 1-800-655-0338* at least one week before the hearing.

Your Right to Review Your Assistance Files: You and/or your representative will be permitted to see your assistance files before the hearing by scheduling an appointment with your eligibility worker in advance of the fair hearing. You or your representative may subpoena witnesses, present evidence, and cross-examine witnesses. The hearing officer must make a decision on all evidence presented at the fair hearing.

Non Discrimination Notice For Recipients: Under federal and state law the Massachusetts Division of Medical Assistance does not discriminate on the basis of race, color, sex, sexual orientation, national origin, religion, creed, age, or handicap. For help with any matter pertaining to this policy, we encourage you to contact the Board of Hearings at *(617) 210-5800 or 1-800-655-0338.*

Complete All Appropriate Sections-Print Clearly

Name of Applicant or Recipient: _____

Address: _____

Telephone No.: _____ Medical Assistance ID or SSN: _____

Cardholder's Name on MassHealth card (if different): _____

I request an interpreter (indicate language _____) to be provided by the Board of Hearings.

Signature: _____ Date: _____

My authorized Representative is: _____ Title: _____

Address: _____ Telephone No.: _____

I, _____ , hereby request a fair hearing before a hearing officer at the Board of Hearings. The reason I wish to request a fair hearing is: _____

_____

_____

☐ A. I do not wish to receive assistance during the appeal process.

☐ B. I request an expedited hearing because: _____

_____

Instructions to *Long Term Care Providers*

The following instructions correspond with numbered items on the reverse side. Please note: For SSI recipients, a copy of the SC-1 must be sent to the appropriate Social Security District Office.

1. Enter today's date, the recipient's region, local welfare office number, category of assistance, and name (please print).

2. Enter the name, address, and phone number of the facility submitting this form.

3. Enter the seven-digit provider number.

4. Enter the date of admission.

5. Enter the date from which Medicaid payment is requested.

6. Enter the appropriate code: A for admitted, D for discharged, or R for both admitted and discharged.

7. Enter the recipient's 10-digit Medicaid identification number, if known.

ITEMS 8 THROUGH 12 ARE FOR INTERNAL MEDICAID USE ONLY

13. Enter the discharge date for the current discharge and if both admitting and discharging.

14. Enter the date of death, if applicable.

15. Use this space to enter any comments.

16. Check box 16A to indicate a short-term stay (6 months or less), 16B to indicate a long-term stay, or 16C to indicate that the short-term stay is terminated and is now long term. Check 16D if the recipient is Medicare eligible upon admission.

17. Enter where recipient is admitted from (i.e., home, name of acute or chronic hospital).

18. Enter where recipient is discharged to (i.e., home, name and address of acute or chronic hospital).

19. Enter the expected length of stay only if the expected stay is six months or less.

20. The physician must sign and date only if the expected stay is six months or less. For a long-term stay, no signature is required.

21. An authorized representative of the facility must sign and date this form.

Commonwealth of Massachusetts
Division of Medical Assistance

Status Change for Recipient in a Long Term Care Facility or Rest Home
(Admission or Discharge of MA or SSI Recipient)

Check Appropriate Box(es)

- 15A. Short term (6 months or less) ☐
- 15B. Long term (more than 6 months) ☐
- 15C. Short-term care stay terminated Now long-term care ☐
- 15D. Medicare upon admission ☐

17. Admitted from: _____

18. Discharged to: _____

Complete Items 19 and 20 Only If Stay is Six Months or Less

19. I certify that the above-named recipient's expected length of stay is _____ (Length of Stay)

20. _____ (Physician's Signature)

Date: _____

21. Signature of Authorized Representative Completing this Form

Date: _____

NOTE: NURSING HOME SCREENING NOTIFICATION FORM OR ADMISSION DETERMINATION LETTER MUST BE ATTACHED.

1. Date ____ Reg ____ LWO ____ Cat ____

Recipient's Name ____ Last ____ First ____ MI ____

2. Name of Facility Submitting this Notification

Name: _____ Address: _____ Phone: _____

3. Provider Number _____

4. Admit Date _____

5. Recipient ID/SSN _____

7. Recipient ID/SSN _____

6. ☐ A - Admit ☐ D - Discharge ☐ R - Both Admit and Discharge

FOR DIVISION USE ONLY

8. PPA Amount ____ Eff. Date (MM/YY) ____ Retro PPA ☐

Eff. Date (MM/YY) ____ ☐

9. Level of Care ____ 10. MA Start Date ____

11. Discharge Reason ____ 12. Worker CAN ____

13. Discharge Date _____

14. Date of Death _____

15. Comments: _____

SEE REVERSE FOR INSTRUCTIONS FOR COMPLETION OF THIS FORM.

SC-1 (Rev. 2/94)

Chapter 9:
Conclusion

This Handbook is designed to assist very special people: those who are willing to step up and help a vulnerable population: frail elders who are not only sick, but unable to cope mentally and financially with their current lot in life. Anyone willing to serve as a guardian for an indigent nursing home resident should be able to get whatever help, guidance, and assistance needed to do the job well.

The nursing home system will be better and safer as more and more guardians take their places as integral parts of the healthcare system, which we hope will treat us all fairly and competently. Guardians will not only assure the rights of incapacitated nursing home residents, they will also improve the quality of life in the long-term care system as they help nursing home staff, ombudsmen, and DPH surveyors to meet their goal of seeing that the system works well for all.

A guardian should not be reluctant to ask for help as the demands of the task undertaken become greater when the needs of the ward increase or become emergencies. Even well trained and experienced guardians find the job demanding and ask for help when needed.

A guardian should organize the affairs of the ward and maintain good medical and financial records. Maintaining a journal is a good idea, and using a checklist like the one at the end of this Chapter will help keep the guardian's thoughts organized, and make things run more smoothly.

A guardian should not be reluctant to seek counsel on issues grand and small. If the ward cannot help with information about his or her wishes regarding medical care, there may be other sources whom the guardian can consult: relatives, friends, or associates. At all times, the guardian must use the ward's values when deciding medical issues, whether they relate to minor treatment, surgeries, participation in research projects or studies, organ donations, Alzheimer's research involving the post-mortem study of the patient's brain, or any other issue. The guardian's decisions must be informed by the perennial question: What would be the ward's wishes if she or he could understand the situation and speak to me about those wishes? That is the challenge of the guardian: To enable the ward to enjoy life to the best of his or her capability and according to his or her own wishes.

GUARDIAN'S CHECKLIST: _____

Name of Guardian

_____

Name of Ward

_____

Social Security Number

_____

Date of Birth

Date prepared:

The records and important documents of the ward are stored in one of the following locations:

(A)

(B)

(C)

Item

Guardianship appointment: decree of court _____

Birth certificate _____

Marriage certificate _____

Durable power of attorney document (original) _____

Health care proxy document (original) _____

Last will and testament (original) _____

Life insurance policy/policies _____

Health insurance policy/policies _____

Nursing Home care plan _____

Funeral contract/trust   _____

Deed(s) to real estate   _____

Military/veteran's documents   _____

List of bank accounts   _____

Retirement papers   _____

Pension information   _____

Motor vehicle title documents   _____

List of creditors   _____

Credit card statements   _____

List of family, friends   _____

List of stored or loaned items   _____

List of treating physicians   _____

List of medications   _____

Records re: business income   _____

Records re: Spouse or children   _____

Other: _____

Emergency contacts:

Doctor   _____

Clergy   _____

Attorney   _____

Accountant   _____

Insurance agent   _____

Other: _____

Resources

Table of Contents

AGING SERVICES ACCESS POINTS (ASAPS)

Aging Service Access Points are non-profit agencies that provide services, information, and referrals to elders and their advocates. Among their responsibilities is the job of evaluating an individual to determine whether he or she meets the medical criteria for admission or continued stay at a nursing home. Their Information and Referral services are excellent resources.

There are 28 ASAP's in the Commonwealth.

ALZHEIMER'S ASSOCIATION

The Alzheimer's Association is a nation-wide organization devoted to serving Alzheimer's patients and their families in a wide range of areas: information and referral, advocacy, public policy, and medical research.

Alzheimer's Association, Massachusetts Chapter

36 Cameron Street

Cambridge, MA 02140

617-868-6718 or www.alzmass.org

Help line: 1-800-548-2111

ATTORNEY GENERAL'S OFFICE

The Massachusetts Attorney General's office has a number of duties and functions that may impact a nursing home resident. The AG staff may respond to complaints that a nursing home has violated the consumer protection laws or regulations (940 C.M.R. 4.00) or any other laws of the Commonwealth. The Attorney General, for example, prosecutes Medicaid fraud (criminal) matters that may involve very serious matters such as physical harm or the death of a resident. District Attorneys in each county also prosecute criminal matters.

Attorney General

One Ashburton Place, 20th floor

Boston, MA 02108

617-727-2200 or www.ago.state.ma.us

Elder Citizens Service Hotline (888- 243-5337)

Consumer Protection Hotline (617-727-8400)

Public Protection Bureau (617-727-2200)

DEPARTMENT OF PUBLIC HEALTH

The Massachusetts Department of Public Health licenses nursing homes, monitors the quality of the health care received by residents (by means of surveyors, inspectors, and complaint investigators) and presides over the closing of a nursing home.

Department of Public Health

250 Washington Street

Boston, MA 02108-5220

617-624-6000

Legal Division

Division of Health Care Quality (surveyors) 617-753-8000

Complaints (report of abuse)

Bureau of Health Quality Management (nursing home "report cards")

ELDER LEGAL SERVICES PROGRAMS

There are a number of free legal services programs that serve low-income and elderly residents of Massachusetts. The services are funded by grants mostly from the Massachusetts Legal Assistance Corporation, the Area Agencies on Aging (Title III of the federal Older Americans Act funds), the National Legal Services Corporation, the Massachusetts Bar Foundation, and other supporters. There is a legal services web site at www.MassLegalServices.org. Click on **Find Legal Services** to locate the legal service agency serving the city or town where the resident lives.

Massachusetts Legal Assistance Corporation (MLAC)

11 Beacon Street, Suite 820

Boston, MA 02108

617-367-8544 or www.MassLegalServices.org

(MLAC does not provide legal services but funds state-wide and local programs that do so.)

The elder services programs funded to serve elders, age 60 and over are:

EXECUTIVE OFFICE OF ELDER AFFAIRS

The Massachusetts Executive Office of Elder Affairs (E.O.E.A.) has as its mission to serve the needs of elders in the Commonwealth. The E.O.E.A. distributes federal and state funds to support the work of the ASAP's, elder protective services and elders at risk, the nursing home ombudsman programs, home care services, Councils on Aging, and SHINE volunteers.

Executive Office of Elder Affairs

One Ashburton Place, 5th floor

Boston, MA 02108

617-727-7750

Tel: 1-800-AGE-INFO

State Nursing Home Ombudsman

Protective Services

SHINE (Serving the Health Insurance Needs of Elders) counselors

MASSHEALTH ENROLLMENT CENTERS

Long-term care Medicaid applications are filed at one of four regional offices of the Division of Medical Assistance:

MEC

21 Spring Street, Suite 4

Taunton, MA 02780

Tel: 508-828-4600 (1-800-242-1340)

MEC

300 Ocean Avenue, Suite 4000

Revere, MA 02151

Tel: 781-485-2500 (1-800-322-1448)

MEC

367 East Street

Tewksbury, MA 01876

Tel: 978-863-9200 (1-800-408-1253)

MEC

333 Bridge Street

Springfield, MA 01103

Tel: 413-785-4100 (1-800-332-5545)

MEDEX (MEDIGAP INSURANCE)

The most common form of MediGap insurance (covering the co-pays and deductibles of Medicare coverage) is the Blue Cross Blue Shield operated Medex program. Questions may be directed to BC/BS or to a SHINE counselor.

Blue Cross Blue Shield of Massachusetts

Tel: 1-800-451-8124 or www.bluecrossma.com

MEDICARE

Medicare insurance may cover some nursing home costs. Although Medicare appeals may end up in the Social Security Administration's Office of Hearings and Appeals, claims and low-level appeals are administered by the insurance intermediary. Medicare maintains a web site to inform consumers of the performance of nursing homes according to surveys or inspections done.

Nursing Home Care Compare 1-800- 633-4227 or www.medicare.gov

NATIONAL ACADEMY OF ELDER LAW ATTORNEYS—MASSACHU-SETTS. CHAPTER

The National Academy of Elder Law Attorneys is a national association of elder law practitioners. The Massachusetts Chapter has members all over the state and will make referrals.

Mass NAELA

P.O. Box 67137

Chestnut Hill, MA 02467

Tel: 617-566-56430 or www.manaela.org

NURSING HOME OMBUDSMAN PROGRAMS

Nursing home ombudsman programs are found throughout the Commonwealth and are typically located in an ASAP. To contact a local ombudsman program, either call the local ASAP or the State Nursing Home Ombudsman at the E.O.E.A. offices

PROBATE COURTS

Probate Courts are located in each county:

PUBLICATIONS

A Guide for Elders: Planning that Protects You and Your Assets

Published by the Gerontology Institute and available on line:

www.geront.umb.edu ; Click on **Literature**; Click on **Resources and Information for Older Persons**; Click on **Guide for Elders**.

Guide to Long-Term Care Alternatives in Massachusetts

VA/DEPARTMENT OF VETERANS SERVICES

There are federal and state programs for veterans. Eligibility for benefits or services vary, depending on income, years of military services, disability, military service-connected disability, or relationship to a veteran. Most cities and towns have veterans service officers, and there are several veterans organizations that offer advocacy services to veterans.

Department of Veterans Affairs (federal)

JFK Federal Building

Boston, MA

617-565-2599

Department of Veterans Services (state)

239 Causeway Street, Suite 100

Boston, MA 02114

617-727-3578

Soldiers Homes: Chelsea 617-884-5660

Holyoke 413-532-9475

MISCELLANEOUS

Gerontology Institute, University of Massachusetts Boston, 617-287-7300 or www.geront.umb.edu

Massachusetts Commission for the Blind: 1-800-392-6450

Massachusetts Commission for the Deaf: 1-800-223-2559

Social Security Administration: 1-800-772-1213 www.ssa.gov

Glossary

AAAs Area Agencies on Aging are organizations designated by the federal Administration on Aging (AoA) to receive federal grant funds to serve the needs of elders in the greatest social and economic need. Typically, they fund elder nutrition programs, transportation, day care, and legal services. In Massachusetts, most AAAs are ASAPs, that is, not-for-profit corporations set up to serve the elder population in their catchment areas. For a list of the ASAPs/AAAs, call 1-800-AGE-INFO.

ADLs Actiities of daily living is a term used in the elder care network to describe normal everyday activities that frail or incapacitated persons may need assistance in performing. Those activities are: bathing, dressing, feeding, toileting, transferring (e.g., from bed to chair), ambulating. Medicaid uses this term in describing the criteria for placement in a nursing home, by mandating that a resident requires assistance with a specific number of ADLs as well as with skilled nursing care.

affidavit of indigency A sworn statement filed with the court that asserts under pains and penalties of perjury that the party is indigent and entitled to proceed without having to pay court costs or fees. Massachusetts law permits an indigent person to access the court pursuant to G.L. c. 261 §§ 27A—27G . For a sample Affidavit of Indigency, see Appendix 6-B.

annuity The right to receive annual or other periodic payment as a result of having purchased an annuity contract with the payment of a lump sum. To understand why annuities may be important, see the answer to Question 24 in Chapter 7.

anti-psychotic medication	Medications used to treat psychoses or the more severe symptoms of dementia. A Rogers guardianship is required when a patient lacks the capacity to give informed consent to the administration of such medications and has not designated in writing a healthcare proxy agent who can authorize such treatment. For a list of the current medications considered to be anti-psychotic, see Appendix 6-A1.
appeal	The review of a decision at the request of a person aggrieved by that decision by an authority greater than the original decision maker. An applicant who is denied Medicaid coverage by a worker can appeal to the DMA Board of Hearings and appeal further to the Superior Court for judicial review of the decision.
appellant	A person seeking the review of a decision by a greater authority.
assessment (medical)	An evaluation of the medical needs of a person who is about to be admitted or is already admitted to a nursing home, to determine whether Medicaid will contribute to the costs of that person's care. Currently, the medical criteria is that the person must require at least one skilled nursing care need and require assistance with at least two ADLs. This is the so-called "Score three" test.
assessment (spousal assets)	The determination by Medicaid, at the time of application for long-term care coverage, as to which of the marital assets are considered to be those of the community spouse and which are considered to be those of the institutionalized spouse. Any assets of the latter must be spent down for his/her care to the $2000 allowable limit. See the answer to Question 9 in Chapter 7.
asset allowance	The amount of marital assets which Medicaid considers available either to the institutionalized spouse or to the community spouse.

assets (resources)	Real or personal property that will be part of the review of an applicant's eligibility for long-term care Medicaid. Assets can be countable or non-countable, depending on their nature and accessibility.
ASAP	Aging Systems Access Points are non-profit corporations that provide services, information, and referrals to elders residing in Massachusetts. There are 28 such organizations throughout the Commonwealth, and they are listed in the Resources section of this handbook. Many ASAPs are AAAs.
autonomy	Self-determination, free from the control of others.
bed hold	A term applied to Medicaid's payment to "hold" a nursing home bed when the resident is on "medical leave of absence," that is, hospitalized. Currently, Medicaid requires a nursing home to hold a Medicaid eligible resident's bed for up to 10 days while a nursing home resident is being treated for an acute illness in a hospital. There is no payment by Medicaid to the facility while the bed is being held.
Brophy guardianship	Refers to a guardianship proceeding relative to a patient who is in a persistent vegetative state and where the court's inquiry considers whether the patient, if able to speak, would authorize or decline life supports.
case manager	One who coordinates the providers of medical and social services to an elder.
CFR	Code of Federal Regulations. These are regulations promulgated by federal agencies, like the Social Security Administration or the Center for Medicare and Medicaid Services (CMS), to implement their programs, outline their responsibilities, and set out the rights of any beneficiaries under their programs. For example, 42 C.F.R. § 483.12 describes what a nursing home must do when transferring or discharging a resident.

community spouse   A married person whose spouse is a nursing home resident or in a hospital when he or she is no longer acutely ill but awaiting a nursing home placement.

community spouse
resource allowance   That portion of marital assets that Medicaid says the community spouse is allowed to keep for his or her financial needs in the process of determining whether a nursing home spouse is eligible for Medicaid coverage. See Questions 9 and 10 in Chapter 7.

CMR   Code of Massachusetts Regulations. These are regulations promulgated by state agencies to implement their programs, outline their responsibilities, and set out the rights of any beneficiaries under their programs. For example, 106 C.M.R. 520.026(E)(3) describes how the guardian of a nursing home resident may be reimbursed for expenses and compensated for the guardianship services provided. Because of this regulations's significance to the subject matters of this Handbook, the regulation is found in its entirety in Appendix 6-O.

CMS   Center for Medicare and Medicaid Services. The federal agency responsible for overseeing the operations of the Medicare and Medicaid programs. The CMS monitors the state's Medicaid operations as well as the medical providers who treat or care for Medicare- and Medicaid- eligible persons.

CNA   Certified Nursing Assistant, a term used to describe a particular nursing home staffer. DPH regulations at 105 C.M.R. 156.020 define a CNA as "any individual who provides nursing care under the supervision of a nurse in a long-term care facility."

confidentiality   The right of an individual to have information kept privileged or secret and not released to anyone without the express consent of the individual.

conflict of interest   This term describes a situation where a person in a fiduciary capacity has conflicting loyalties between two persons or entities. For example, a person who will benefit financially if a ward's resources are saved rather than spent on his or her care may be in a conflict of interest sufficient to be disqualified to serve as a guardian.

conservator

Sometimes referred to as "guardian of the estate," a conservator is a Probate Court appointed fiduciary responsible for managing the financial affairs, but not the personal or medical affairs, of the ward.

consumer
price index

Statistics published by the U.S. Department of Labor that tracks such topics as consumer price increase and poverty levels based on the costs of living in the various regions of the nation. Poverty level figures are significant for a number of reasons, including the impact on a community spouse's right to keep marital assets or a spouse's income to bring his or her actual income up to meet 150% of the federal poverty level for two persons, in order to avoid impoverishment.

convalescent
home

Also referred to as a rest home, a residential facility that is distinguishable from a skilled nursing facility (nursing home) in that it does not have available to residents around the clock medical care, but rather supportive services (meals, cleaning, linen service, cuing for medications). Sometimes referred to as a Level IV facilities, they are considerably less expensive than nursing homes and are largely disappearing in the wake of newer (and more expensive) assisted living programs

Council on Aging

Nearly every city and town in Massachusetts has a Council on Aging, whose primary function is to assist elderly persons with information about and referral to services available to that population. For a complete list of COA's, call 1-800-AGE-INFO.

countable assets

See "assets."

CSIA

Community spouse income allowance is a Medicaid term that refers to the amount of the institutionalized spouse's monthly income that the community spouse is entitled to retain in order for him or her to avoid impoverishment. A CSIA will permit the community spouse to have income up to his or her MMMNA, which is 150% of the Federal Poverty Level for two persons, with an potential adjustment for excessive shelter costs. See Question 10 in Chapter 7 for a complete discussion.

CSRA   Community spouse resource allowance is a Medicaid term referring to the amount of marital assets that the community spouse is allowed to retain for his or her use. See answers to Questions 9 and 10 in Chapter 7.

de facto guardian   A person who acts or is treated by medical providers as if he or she has authority to act as the guardian of another person when no such authority exists in the law.

de iure guardian   A person who has the authority to act as the guardian of another person, by virtue of having been appointed by the Probate Court to exercise such authority.

dementia   Deterioration of mental faculties like memory and judgment, usually accompanied by emotional disturbance. Not a diagnosis, dementia can have many causes, and is not necessarily irreversible. A guardian should oblige the medical providers to perform tests to determine whether a ward's dementia is reversible.

determination of eligibility   An income program such as Social Security or SSI or a medical health coverage program like Medicare or Medicaid have rules of eligibility. The eligibility may be based on a work record (Social Security-Medicare) or financial need (SSI-Medicaid) but in every case an application must be filed to establish entitlement to benefits and the agency administering the program reviews the application and makes a determination of eligibility based on the rules of each program.

disability trust   There are special Medicaid and SSI rules relative to trusts established for disabled individuals. Any issue involving the rights of a ward under a trust or the right to establish a trust for the ward should be reviewed with a trust or elder law attorney.

discharges (and transfers)

A term referring to a nursing home's action to remove a resident from a facility. A transfer implies a temporary move where the nursing home is not terminating its obligation to care for the resident but rather is recommending a move based on the need for care not available at the facility, most often a transfer to a hospital for treatment of an acute illness. A discharge implies that the nursing home seeks to terminate its obligation to care for the resident and does not want to re-admit the resident once removed. The nursing home's authority to transfer or discharge residents involuntarily is strictly monitored. See Question 17 in Chapter 2.

discharge of guardianship

The process by which a ward who has recovered his or her capacity to manage him- or herself and his or her affairs can have the Probate Court discharge or dissolve the guardianship. A guardian may also be discharged or removed for cause.

DMA

Division of Medical Assistance (also known as Medicaid and Mass Health), the agency responsible for administering the state/federal partnership program for medical care for eligible persons known as Medicaid.

DMA enrolment centers

The enrollment centers are where the DMA conducts its business, accepting and processing applications, reviews, hearings, and so on. For a complete list of the enrollment centers, see the Resources section.

DPH

Department of Public Health is a state agency responsible for licensing of long-term care facilities and for monitoring the quality of the care provided residents. Among its more significant functions are the periodic surveys (inspections) of facilities and its complaint investigation unit. DPH-related information can be found in the Resources section.

DTA   Department of Transitional Assistance, which provides income assistance to families whose income falls below the income standards for the program.

due process   This term applies to the exercise of power or authority as the laws dictate, with appropriate respect for the individual rights of parties seeking entitlements from those exercising that authority. So, officials of the DMA, for example, must follow their own rules and regulations as they process an individual's application for assistance throughout the administrative process. Any decision can be appealed, with the burden on the appellant to demonstrate that the decision being appealed is contrary to the governing rules.

durable power
of attorney   A written document by which an individual (the principal) gives or grants to an "attorney in fact" (or agent) the legal authority to manage that individual's personal, financial, or other matters in the event that the individual is absent, incapacitated, or otherwise unable to manage those affairs him- or herself. See Chapter 2, *Guide for Elders,* on the UMass Boston Gerontology Institute's web site at www.geront.umb.edu, click on Literature. Then, click on Resources and Information for Older Persons, and then on Guide for Elders.

DVS   The Department of Veterans Affairs, which is a state-funded program for veterans and their dependents and survivors. For more information on the DVS, see the Resources section.

EAEDC   Emergency Assistance to Elders, Disabled, and Children is a state program of income assistance for very low-income persons who qualify financially for such assistance. The EAEDC program pays a subsidy to rest homes for any SSI- or EAEDC-eligible resident, since Medicaid does not subsidize rest home care.

eligibility	Entitlement to receive income, goods, or services, pursuant to the rules of an entitlement programs, for example, the Medicaid program.
EOEA	Executive Office of Elder Affairs. See the Resources section for more information.
estate recovery	In Medicaid parlance, estate recovery refers to the right of the Medicaid program to recover from the estate of a deceased Medicaid enrollee all of the costs incurred by Medicaid on behalf of that enrollee during his or her lifetime while receiving Medicaid coverage. In 2003, the definition of estate was expanded to include any property interest held by the deceased Medicaid recipient at the time of his or her death. See answer to Question 16 in Chapter 7.
extraordinary treatment	This term applies to a guardianship proceeding where the ward is alleged to need out-of-the-ordinary medical treatment, for example, life supports (*Brophy* cases) or anti-psychotic medications (*Rogers* cases). The guardian must request authority from the court to permit extraordinary treatment.
facility	*See* "Levels of care."
fair hearing	The DMA is required by federal and state law to permit any person aggrieved of a decision by a worker to conduct a fair hearing to review the appeal filed by that aggrieved person. Appeals must be filed with the Board of Hearings within the time permitted (usually 30 days) and are conducted by independent hearing officers who take evidence and issue a written ruling that can be further appealed and reviewed by the Superior Court. See discussion at the end of Chapter 8.
fiduciary responsibility	A fiduciary is one who holds a position of trust with respect to another person or his or her property, and the relationship is one of trust and requires scrupulous good faith, honesty, loyalty, and candor.

FPL   Federal Poverty Level.

guardian
ad litem   Guardian ad litem (GAL) is an individual appointed by the Probate Court to investigate the circumstances of a case, interview parties and witnesses, review relevant documents such as medical records, and make a report back to the court. GALs are used largely to expedite court proceedings; such appointments may result in parties' not having to wait a long period of time for the always busy courts to conduct full hearings when a GAL may be able to resolve the matter between the parties or at least narrow the issues in dispute.

**geriatric care
specialist**   A professional advocate who has extensive knowledge and experience in the elder care and healthcare systems and is available to assist in planning for the healthcare needs of elders.

guardian   An individual appointed by the Probate Court to manage the affairs of another, called a Ward.

guardianship   The state of one's having another person in control of one's affairs.

HCP law   The healthcare proxy law establishes the guidelines by which every adult person may sign a written document granting authority to a person of their choice to make healthcare decisions when the grantor is incapable of giving informed consent to any proposed medical treatment. The law, found at M.G.L. c. 201D, is discussed in the *Guide for Elders*, available on the UMass Gerontology website at www.geront.umb.edu. Then, click on **Literature** and then on **Resources and Information for Older Persons**, then on **Guide for Elders**.

**healthcare
proxy agent**   A person appointed in a written document signed by the principal and witnessed by two persons, who will exercise authority to make health care and medical decisions for the principal when the treating physician

and the agent agree that the principal no longer has the capacity to make such decisions.

healthcare proxy document The document by which the person signing grants authority to a person of their choice to make health care decisions when the grantor is incapable of giving informed consent to any proposed medical treatment.

HMO Health Maintenance Organizations, which manage the healthcare of its enrollees and have been touted as being more efficient vehicles for providing healthcare.

home care services Medical, health, or social services furnished in one's home by nurses, home health aides, housekeepers, personal care attendants, etc.

hospice care Hospice care describes the kind of medical care and treatment to be furnished to terminally ill patients. Generally, the care is palliative, designed to make the patient as comfortable as possible, rather than curative.

inaccessible asset A Medicaid term referring to an asset that would ordinarily be counted as a resource for an applicant or recipient in determining eligibility, but is not counted because the resource is unavailable and cannot be used for the person's healthcare needs.

incapacitated Lacking the ability or capacity to do or perform certain activities.

income first rule A Medicaid term describing one manner in which Medicaid can treat the income and assets of a married couple when one spouse is in a nursing home. Unlike the assets first rule, the income first rule greatly disadvantages low-income community spouses by reducing the availability of marital asset to avoid the impoverishment of community spouses. See answers to Questions 10 in Chapter 7.

incompetent A term still applied in guardianship proceedings to describe a ward's inability to manage him- or herself or his or her affairs. A legal rather than medical term, it is largely criticized for its vagueness, with many legal and medical professionals preferring to use the term "incapacitated."

informed consent

Informed consent is the legal requirement that a patient must authorize any medical treatment being proposed and is based on the patient's understanding of the medical condition being treated and of the risks and benefits of the proposed treatment.

institutionalized spouse

The member of a married couple admitted to or about to be admitted to a skilled nursing care facility

institutionalized spouse resource allowance

The amount of marital assets considered by Medicaid to be available for the use of the institutionalized spouse and which must be spent down to the permissible level of $2000 before eligibility for long-term care Medicaid can be established.

intestate

The legal term used to describe a person who dies without leaving a valid last will and testament. In such cases, state law determines who shares in the estate. See Appendix 6-A1 (Law of Intestate Succession).

insurance: cash surrender value

The value that can be obtained from a whole life insurance policy if it were to be returned to the insurer for its current or cash value, the insured still being alive.

insurance: face value

The value obtained from a life insurance policy by the beneficiary from the insurer upon the death of the insured.

irrevocable funeral trust

A pre-need funeral contract and trust that is established with a funeral director and that is permitted by Medicaid to the extent that funds in such a trust are not countable assets. Medicaid even permits the funding of such a trust from assets that have been held countable as a permissible use of the funds.

irrevocable trust   A trust established by a trustor (sometimes called a settlor), the terms of which may not be changed or revoked.

judicial review   Review by the Superior Court of any action taken by state agencies, like the DMA, pursuant to M.G.L. c. 30A. A plaintiff appellant does not get a full trial hearing on such an appeal but rather must show to the court that the DMA hearing officer committed an error of law or otherwise abused his or her authority.

levels of care   This term refers to the nature of long-term care facilities licensed by the DPH. Although the terms are outdated, their use persists. **Level I** refers to medical care of the highest (long-term care) level where the resident requires daily skilled nursing care; it is often used to describe care paid for by Medicare. **Levels II and III** refer to daily skilled nursing care not paid for by Medicare (**II**) and care involving some nursing care but not delivered daily and also care in the form of assistance with ADLs (**III**). **Level IV** refers to rest homes that are medical facilities in that nurses are not available full time, and Medicaid does not pay for such care. See answer to Question 12 in Chapter 4 for a discussion of rest home reimbursement.

liens   A security interest in real estate, filed in the County Registry of Deeds and by which the lien holder assures payment of a debt. A mortgage is the typical lien. The DMA may place a notice lien on real estate of a recipient to ensure estate recovery or earlier payment if the real estate is sold while the recipient is still alive. See answer to Question 23 in Chapter 7 for a discussion of DMA liens.

limited guardianship   A guardianship established by the Probate Court that is not "plenary," or full, but rather has limits established on the guardian's authority. A court has extensive authority to set guidelines or limits for the guardian. For example, a court may order that the ward may not be admitted to a mental health facility or a nursing home without the prior approval of the court.

living trust

A trust which is revocable. Assets in such a trust avoid probate, but not the creditors of a deceased person who has established such a trust. Medicaid will consider assets in a revocable trust as available (countable) for an applicant who created the trust even if the trust asset in the trust is an ordinarily non-countable asset like the applicant's principal residence. In such a case, the trust will have to be revoked before eligibility can be established.

living will

A document by which an individual indicates his or her wishes with respect to extraordinary medical care, such as life support systems like the use of an artificial respirator or feeding tubes, for the guidance of medical providers in the event that the individual is unable to express such wishes. Living wills are not recognized in Massachusetts, and even a living will lawfully executed in a state outside Massachusetts will not necessarily avoid the need for a Brophy guardianship. Healthcare proxy documents executed pursuant to M.G.L. c. 201D permit the writer to give instructions to his or her agent regarding how to deal with such issues. See healthcare proxy, above.

long-term care

Care furnished to a person with chronic illness or medical conditions, provided in a variety of environments, from the individual's home through the spectrum of elder housing, foster care, congregate living, assisted living, rest home, nursing home, and chronic care hospitals.

LTC insurance

Long-term care insurance covers the insured for some of the costs of long-term care. Historically, it has been criticized for being either too costly for good coverage or lacking good coverage to the extent of its affordability. A significant advantage to buying long-term care insurance is that a person who has long-term care insurance (of particular coverage amounts) on the day of admission to a nursing home avoids any Medicaid estate recovery, regardless of how long his or her stay is covered by a Medicaid subsidy.

MassHealth   *See* "**Medicaid.**"

MCCA   The Medicare Catastrophic Coverage Act of 1988, a federal law that made significant changes to how Medicare and Medicaid pay for long-term care expenses.

MEDEX   The most common form of MediGap insurance, that is, health insurance that covers gaps in Medicare insurance coverage.

Medicaid   A program that pays for healthcare and medical costs for low-income individuals who qualify under all rules of the program. Medicaid subsidizes the costs of care of some 75% of all nursing home residents in Massachusetts.

2. Medicaid-eligible   A Medicaid-eligible person is one who has been approved for coverage of the costs of all covered services furnished by medical providers who participate in the Medicaid system.

Medicare   Federal health and medical insurance that accompanies eligibility for regular (not early) Social Security retirement or Social Security disability benefits after the insured has been receiving such benefits for two years.

Medication (anti-psychotic)   *See* "**anti-psychotic medications.**"

MediGap insurance   Health insurance that covers gaps in Medicare insurance coverage.

MMMNA   Minimum Monthly Maintenance Needs Allowance is a Medicaid term referring to the right of a community spouse to retain sufficient income to avoid impoverishment by virtue of the nursing home placement of the institutionalized spouse. See answers to Questions 10 and 11 in Chapter 7.

MQT Medicaid Qualifying Trust refers to a Medicaid rule that says that a recipient who established a trust, or whose spouse established a trust, and is entitled, as a beneficiary, to get any income or assets from that trust, is considered to be receiving the maximum payable to him or her as beneficiary, without regard to whether the trustee is actually making any such distributions.

Nominee trust A trust "in name only" in that the person establishing the trust maintains significant control over any property in the trust.

OASDI Old Age Survivors and Disability Insurance, the Social Security income benefits insurance program, funded by payroll deductions, which provides monthly benefits to all who qualify in any of the categories of the title.

OBRA of 1987 The Nursing Home Reform Law, which gave rise to significant protections for nursing home residents, provisions of which are found in various sections of federal statutes.

ombudsman The State Long Term Care Ombudsman Program is operated by the Executive Office of Elder Affairs (E.O.E.A.) and supervises area or local nursing home ombudsman programs that recruit, train, and supervise volunteers who visit nursing homes to ensure quality of life in such facilities by taking and investigating complaints and trying to resolve such problems promptly within the facility.

**patient paid
amount (PPA)**
A Medicaid term that refers to the amount of a nursing home resident's monthly income that he or she must contribute towards the cost of his or her care. See answer to Question 11 in Chapter 7.

**personal needs
account**
An account either maintained at the nursing home or in a bank or financial institution, which represents the accumulated savings of a nursing home resident derived from his personal needs allowance.

**personal needs
allowance**
The amount of a nursing home resident's monthly income that a nursing home resident is permitted to retain for personal needs, haircuts, slippers, magazines, and the like. The amount is currently $65.00 and for veterans and veterans' surviving spouses, $90.00.

**petition to
partition**
A Probate Court proceeding wherein a joint owner of real estate petitions the court to appoint commissioners with authority to sell such real estate and distribute the sale proceeds appropriately.

**plenary
authority**
Full and "unlimited" authority, usually applied to the authority of a guardian and distinguished from that of a limited guardianship.

**presumption of
capacity**
The law in Massachusetts is that every person is presumed competent until a court of law rules him or her to be incompetent. It is a court and not medical authorities that adjudge lack of competence, since it is a legal, not a medical, term.

primary residence
The principal home of a nursing home resident, significant because it is not a countable assets when determining eligibility for Medicaid.

private pay	This term describes how a nursing home resident who is not Medicaid- or Medicare-eligible pays for the nursing home care. The average private pay rate is calculated annually ($244 per day as of November 2003) and is used to compute the period of ineligibility where a Medicaid applicant has made a forbidden transfer of assets.
Probate Court	The court seated in every county of Massachusetts, which has jurisdiction to hear and decide, among other cases, guardianship matters.
pro bono	Pro bono publico is a term applied to the historical practice and tradition of attorneys' providing services without charge to clients who are indigent.
pro se	This term refers to a person who is representing him- or herself in court proceedings.
public guardianship commission	In many states, there is a public guardianship commission responsible for establishing guardianships for indigent persons who are in need of such services and protection. There is no public guardianship commission law in Massachusetts.
reasonable medical accommodation	Persons with disabilities are entitled to reasonable medical accommodation of those disabilities from anyone providing services, such as landlords, restauranteurs, and nursing homes.
redetermination of eligibility	Once a person is found eligible for Medicaid long-term care coverage, there may be an annual redetermination of eligibility, whereby forms and documentation are submitted in which the recipient must show that he or she continues to meet the financial and medical criteria for eligibility.

removal of guardian

A guardian may be removed by the Probate Court, either acting on its own or on the motion of an interested party, when there is a showing that the guardian is guilty of misconduct, neglect of duty, bad character, maladministration of a trust, physical or mental incapacity or other good cause. See M.G.L. c. 210 § 13A, and Appendix 6-R.

resident

One who lives in a nursing home is referred to as a resident, not a patient, because the setting is primarily considered to be the persons's home, and not a medical facility like a hospital.

respondent

The person who is obliged to respond to the petition filed in the Probate Court (in guardianships, sometimes referred to as the "proposed ward").

restraint

A device, whether physical or chemical, which is designed to restrict movement. Long-term care facilities have been required to be "restraint free" since the federal Nursing Home Reform Act of 1987.

rest home

See "**Levels of Care.**"

retroactive eligibility

Public benefits programs like Medicaid may provide coverage or benefits for a period of time even prior to an application, referred to as "retroactive" coverage. A Medicaid applicant may request that eligibility be established for the three-month period prior to the date on which the application is filed. See first page of Chapter 8.

reverse mortgage

A devise by which an elder who is land poor, that is, has substantial equity in his or her home but is having difficulty meeting living expenses, can make an agreement with a lending institution to draw down monthly amounts (loans) that are not repayable until a date certain, upon the sale of the real estate, or after the death of the elder. See answer to Question 6 in Chapter 7.

revocable trust	A written trust under the terms of which the settlor retained or granted another individual authority to amend, revise, or revoke the terms of the trust. *See* "**Living trust**" above.
3. Rogers guardianship	A Rogers guardianship refers to Probate Court proceedings where the ward is alleged to be mentally ill and in need of anti-psychotic medications in the context of a proposed treatment plan.
Rogers monitor	The Rogers guardian is the monitor of the treatment plan and must report to the court periodically when changes occur in the ward's/patient's condition.
Rudow guardianship	A Rudow guardianship refers to the appointment of a guardian for a nursing home resident, when the guardian's expenses and costs are to be paid for out of the income of the resident.
SC-1 form	A document issued by a nursing home to the Medicaid program, which documents the resident's admission and medical screening. See a sample at Appendix 8-I.
score 3	*See* "**Medical assessment.**"
settlor	A person who creates a trust.
skilled nursing facility	*See* "**Levels of Care.**"
spend down	A Medicaid term describing how income or assets greater than what is permissible must be used or depleted in order for an individual to become eligible for coverage.
springing power of attorney	A durable power of attorney document that provides that the agent's authority is established, not when the document is signed but rather when the principal becomes incapacitated. For a good discussion of the topic of durable power of attorney documents, see the *Guide for Elders,* available on the UMass Gerontology

Institute's website at www.geront.umb.edu. Then, click on **Literature** and then on **Resources and Information for Older Persons**, then on **Guide for Elders**.

spousal waiver

This term describes the Medicaid procedure that permits an at-home frail spouse age 60 years or older to become Medicaid-eligible without regard to the income or assets of the other spouse in the same household. The applicant must be appropriate to a nursing home placement and be receiving services from the local ASAP. See the answer to Question 15 in Chapter 7.

snapshot date

The date of the most recent nursing home admission of one spouse, at which point in time the Medicaid program determines the marital assets to assess which assets are attributed to which spouse.

SSI

A needs-based income program administered by the Social Security Administration to provide an income "floor" to disabled, blind, or elderly persons who qualify financially and otherwise meet the rules of eligibility.

substituted judgment

A determination by the court in a guardianship in which the court substitutes itself for the incapacitated person and finds, with as much precision as possible, based on testimony and other evidence, the desires and needs of that person, were they able to communicate their wishes. The court considers factors like the ward's expressed preferences regarding treatment (like health-care proxy documents or other prior written or oral expression of such preferences), the ward's religious values, the impact of the ward's decision on the ward's family, the possibility of adverse side effects, and the prognosis with or without the proposed treatment. See Superintendent of Belchertown State School v. Saikewicz, 373 Mass 728, 370 N.E.2d 417 (1977)

sureties

Persons who express confidence in the integrity of a guardian by guaranteeing to the court that the guardian will be an honest steward.

survey results	Nursing homes are monitored by Department of Pubic Health surveyors who make a comprehensive report of their findings; survey results are public record.
temporary guardian	A guardian who has been appointed by the Probate Court for a ninety day period, which can be extended, usually to deal with some emergency or critical need of the ward.
testate	The legal term used to describe a person who dies leaving a valid last will and testament. In such cases, the will controls how assets are to be distributed to beneficiaries after creditors are satisfied.
transfer	*See* "**discharges (and transfers).**"
transfer of assets	A gift or transfer of title of assets without receiving fair value in return. Some transfers of assets may disqualify an individual from eligibility for Medicaid or SSI benefits.
transfer of assets penalty	A Medicaid term referring to a situation where an applicant has made transfers, that is, given away assets, which triggers a period of ineligibility. The period of ineligibility is computed by dividing the value of the assets transferred by the average cost of one month private pay (Currently the average daily cost is $244, or $7,320) to arrive at the number of months, beginning with the month in which the forbidden transfer occurred, during which the applicant is disqualified from eligibility. Such transfers can be "cured" if the assets are returned to the applicant.
Uniform Health Decisions Act	A uniform law that includes an option for the lawful exercise of authority by a "surrogate" of a medical patient who lacks the capacity to give informed consent to proposed medical treatment and has no healthcare proxy agent or medical guardian. The UHDA has not been enacted in Massachusetts.

UPC

The Uniform Probate Code has been enacted in most states, and Section V has been brought significant, welcome, and long-overdue reform to guardianship laws and procedures. The Legislature in Massachusetts has been considering a version of the UPC for the past several years but has not acted on the bill.

USC

United State Codes are the statutes of the United States as enacted by the Congress and signed into law by the President.

VA

Federal Department of Veterans Affairs.

ward

An individual over whom the Probate Court has appointed a guardian after a showing that the individual lacks the ability to manage him- or herself or his or her affairs because of a mental illness or inability to communicate because of physical incapacity.

About the Author

ATTORNEY JOHN J. FORD is a graduate of Boston University and the Boston University Law School, where he graduated in 1970. He was a Reginald Heber Smith Fellow 1970-1972, as staff attorney for Vermont Legal Aid, Inc. and Neighborhood Legal Services, Inc.(NLS) in Lynn, MA. He has been the director of the Elder Law Project at NLS since 1977.

Mr. Ford has been an instructor at the North Shore Community College Center for Older Adults and at the University of Massachusetts Gerontology Institute, Boston Campus. This Handbook results from the course which he taught there entitled, "The ABC's of Nursing Home Guardianships"; where the designed course work product would be a consumer friendly Handbook which demystifies long term care Medicaid applications and guardianship proceedings. He has written and lectured extensively on elders' rights especially with respect to incapacity and long term care.

His legal practice has been an active one including serving as chief or lead counsel on a number of landmark cases in Massachusetts, most notably in the case of Rudow v. Division of Medical Assistance (Massachusetts Supreme Judicial Court, 1999) a successful challenge to Medicaid's failure to permit nursing home residents to have a medical /remedial deduction for guardianship costs. Others include Brunelle v. Commissioner, Division of Medical Assistance, a challenge to the Mass Medicaid's refusal to recognize its duty to afford an administrative fair hearing to a nursing home resident who sent to a hospital and refused re-admission to the facility; as a result of the lawsuit, Mass Medicaid revised its regulations in April 2002, to provide for fair hearing when such residents refused re-admission to their nursing home. Studley v Commissioner, Division of Medical Assistance (Barnstable Superior Court 2002), Co-counsel with Attorney Brian Barreira, successful challenge of the DMA's failure to employ a rational methodology for determining the average costs of private pay nursing home care in the calculation of the period of ineligibility resulting from forbidden transfers of assets.

Mr. Ford has participated in drafting statutory provisions and major State regulations, including the original State Long term Care Ombudsman statute, the original Medicaid regulations implementing the Medicare Catastrophic Coverage

Act of 1988 (MCCA) and a major re-drafting of the Massachusetts Attorney General regulations promulgated under the consumer protection Laws, G.L. c. 93A, relative to long term care facilities.

He is Chairman Emeritus of the Elder legal Coalition, the former President of the Massachusetts Chapter of the National Academy of Elder Law Attorneys, and the former President of the Board of Directors of the South Boston Community Health Center.

0-595-32714-1